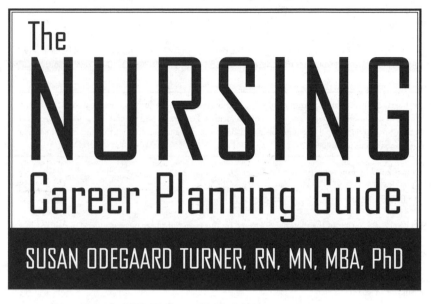

The NURSING
Career Planning Guide

SUSAN ODEGAARD TURNER, RN, MN, MBA, PhD

President/CEO Turner Healthcare Associates, Inc.
Healthcare Advisor, Monster.com

JONES AND BARTLETT PUBLISHERS
Sudbury, Massachusetts
BOSTON   TORONTO   LONDON   SINGAPORE

BP45

World Headquarters

Jones and Bartlett Publishers
40 Tall Pine Drive
Sudbury, MA 01776
978-443-5000
info@jbpub.com
www.jbpub.com

Jones and Bartlett Publishers
Canada
6339 Ormindale Way
Mississauga, Ontario L5V 1J2
CANADA

Jones and Bartlett Publishers
International
Barb House, Barb Mews
London W6 7PA
UK

Jones and Bartlett's books and products are available through most bookstores and online booksellers. To contact Jones and Bartlett Publishers directly, call 800-832-0034, fax 978-443-8000, or visit our website, www.jbpub.com.

Substantial discounts on bulk quantities of Jones and Bartlett's publications are available to corporations, professional associations, and other qualified organizations. For details and specific discount information, contact the special sales department at Jones and Bartlett via the above contact information or send an email to specialsales@jbpub.com.

Copyright © 2007 by Jones and Bartlett Publishers, Inc.
ISBN-13: 978-0-7637-3953-9
ISBN-10: 0-7637-3953-7

Library of Congress Cataloging-in-Publication Data
Turner, Susan Odegaard.
   The nursing career planning guide / Susan Odegaard Turner.
      p. ; cm.
   Includes bibliographical references and index.
   ISBN-13: 978-0-7637-3953-9
   ISBN-10: 0-7637-3953-7
   1. Nursing—Vocational guidance.
   [DNLM: 1. Nursing. 2. Vocational Guidance. 3. Career Choice. 4. Career Mobility. WY 16 T952na 2006] I. Title.
   RT82.T89 2006
   610.7306'9--dc22
                              2006000249
6048

Production Credits
Acquisitions Editor: Kevin Sullivan
Production Director: Amy Rose
Associate Editor: Amy Sibley
Editorial Assistant: Lisa Gordon
Associate Production Editor: Alison Meier
Senior Marketing Manager: Emily Ekle
Manufacturing Buyer: Amy Bacus
Composition: Paw Print Media
Cover Design: Kristin E. Ohlin
Cover Images: © Alamy Images; © Photos.com
Printing and Binding: Malloy, Inc.
Cover Printing: Malloy, Inc.

Printed in the United States of America
10 09 08 07 06   10 9 8 7 6 5 4 3 2 1

10|07|08

Dedication

To Angela and Jordan,
my incredible children.
You are my best life accomplishments!

"For us who Nurse,
Our Nursing is a thing,
Which, unless we are making
Progress every year,
every month, every week …
we are going back."

Florence Nightingale, 1872

Contents

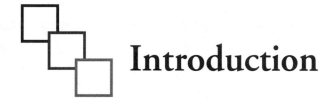

Introduction

This guide was developed to assist nurses at all stages of their careers. The needs of a new graduate nurse are much different than a nurse in her 50s giving up bedside care for less physically demanding work or contemplating retirement. However, issues for nurses are similar, no matter their age or career phase. This book provides information and resources, allowing nurses to make their own choices. It is a book about self-help but also about insight into career decisions.

I am an independent nurse consultant, which allows me to have many different roles. As a consultant, I am a planner, educator, lecturer, writer, mentor, coach, preceptor, and advisor. I use my nursing soul in all these roles. I am also the healthcare career expert for Monster.com. In that career advisory role, I am constantly being asked about nursing as a career and how to deal with issues in the nursing workforce. I am passionate about nursing and extremely proud of being a nurse. I believe that mentoring and coaching other nurses is part of my responsibility as a professional nurse and a way to be of service. I wanted to write a book that would answer the questions I have had throughout my career. I also wanted to share what I learned—both good and bad—about navigating my career. As you move through various stages of your career, you will face different issues. Use this book as part of your career toolkit.

While I am not trained specifically as a career advisor, I believe I have learned things in my 30 years as a nurse that may be useful for others. In writing this book, I have learned that how you manage your nursing career is closely entwined with how you live your life. Self-direction, self-confidence, spiritual connection in daily life and career development are all part of the same continuum. I hope you find this book helpful.

Susan Odegaard Turner

Acknowledgments

Patty Alley—for being a wise and compassionate teacher about life.

Beata Lundeen—for reminding me that nursing is about being of service.

Susan Scott—for teaching me how to be a coach and a mentor.

Ron Gutierrez—for reminding me that, as a nurse, everything I do serves as an example of behavior to others.

Deborah Roberts—for reminding me what really matters is what the patient needs.

Dorothea Glatte—for always believing in me.

Patricia McFarland—for demonstrating daily the kind of commitment and compassion that all nurses strive for.

Charles Padilla (deceased)—for recognizing how much nurses contribute to the patient-care experience.

Kevin Sullivan—for his editorial support with this project.

Katheryn Kray—for being the wind beneath my wings.

Chapter 1
Nursing as a Career

"Shoot for the moon. Even if you miss it you will land among the stars."
—LES BROWN

"The future is not predetermined. It is created by individuals who share enthusiasm for tomorrow's alternatives."
—AUTHOR UNKNOWN

Choosing Nursing as a Career

I am a registered nurse, an independent consultant, and educator, as well as the health-care career advisor for Monster.com. On Monster.com message boards, I receive emails every day from people asking about nursing as a career. Readers are interested in what the educational requirements are, how long the nursing program is, how much blood and body fluids they have to deal with, and what the salaries are for new nurses.

First and foremost, it is important to remember that nursing is a service profession. The fundamental roles and tasks in nursing mean being involved, often intimately, with another human being. Many of the emails I receive start out by asking how much money a nurse can expect to earn once out of nursing school. My response is always that money is not the ruler by which to select nursing as a career. Although many nursing roles offer very good salaries, the essence of nursing is about people. As Ophelia Long, RN, BSN, says, "Nursing affords the opportunity to make a difference

1

in the lives of others. You can earn good money, but you can also make a difference" (Hugg, 2005).

Lots of people ask if being a nurse is difficult because you are exposed to blood, feces, and other various unpleasant body fluids. I have yet to meet a nurse who truly enjoys this aspect of our work, but these tasks do not define the art and science of nursing. Nursing is about caring and being present for a stranger. Nursing is the glue that holds hospital care together. Nurses are the choreographers of the patient-care process. Patients wouldn't need to stay in hospitals if they didn't need nursing care. Almost every other function in hospitals can be done in another location. There are many important roles provided by competent professionals in hospitals. However, it is nurses who oversee and provide the care patients need while hospitalized.

Deciding to become a nurse can be a calling for some. I knew when I was four years old that nursing was the profession I wanted to be involved in. I made the decision after being on the scene of a traffic accident. I liked the idea of being present for someone in pain and making them feel better. Lots of folks enter nursing now as a second career and bring their life wisdom from other fields with them. Many others choose nursing as a career because of the flexible hours, job variety, and ability to continue working while raising children.

Empathy and compassion are the foundations of nursing care. There are many complex tasks required in the role, but choosing the profession of nursing is about caring and wanting to be involved with others. It is an honor to be involved in people's most important life moments—birth, death, or surgery. Few jobs allow that sort of intimate connection with another human being throughout life's numerous transitions and experiences. It is important that potential nurses understand this concept prior to going through the logistics to enter a nursing program. Many of the students who quit nursing school before completing the program do so because they don't realize what the role of a professional nurse entails.

I think the nursing profession needs to make absolutely certain that when we recruit folks into nursing, we make sure they realize that nursing is a service industry. Our job is to serve others. Most people recognize that nurses provide caring. But, as paramedic Mike Smith (2005) said so eloquently about being a paramedic:

> There are two different facets to caring. First is the actual provision of care the techniques, therapeutics and technologies that . . . [are employed] for patients. That kind of taking care of people should be polished, honed and refined throughout your career. The second is having a caring attitude. If you truly care about the patients you service, it will be evident. Every aspect of your practice will include a caring touch, and that is something to be proud of. The ongoing cultivation and nurturing of a caring attitude and overall demeanor is yet another facet of moving beyond competency.

This is true for nurses as well. A winning combination for nurses is continually expanding your knowledge of professional practice and skills, having a commitment to serve patients to the best of your ability, and maintaining a caring attitude.

Not all people are able to become nurses or feel the pull to this type of work. If you do choose nursing as a career, it can consume you. You must learn to take care of yourself in order to be balanced enough to provide care to others. You will encounter difficult staff members, angry physicians, and disgruntled family members. You will be exhausted, frustrated, exhilarated, saddened, and profoundly touched by what you see and do. If you choose nursing, you will work hard, cry often, and have endless job options. You will never, ever be disappointed, because you will always make a difference!

With all the media coverage of the deepening nursing shortage, you may wonder if those working as nurses enjoy their work. According to the 2004 National Survey of Registered Nurses (Steefel, 2005), 9 out of 10 nurses are satisfied with nursing as a career, regardless of their position. Most would even recommend a career in nursing. In fact, nurses are more content with their careers in nursing than physicians, teachers, or attorneys, according to this study. The 2002 NurseWeek/AONE National Survey of Registered nurses also indicated high levels of overall satisfaction with nursing careers.

The reasons for this satisfaction are based largely on the organization in which the nurse works. How loyal a nurse feels to an organization depends on relationships with colleagues and managers. Positive relationships with managers as well as job security, salary and benefits, and the ability to balance work and family all contribute to nurses' job and career satisfaction. Nurses who are recognized for their accomplishments and have a chance to influence decision-making are those most satisfied with their careers.

One of the biggest frustrations, identified in both these studies as well as others, is the inordinate number of non-nursing tasks that nurses must do to make patient systems work. Feeling overburdened by these non-nursing tasks has a negative impact on nurses' perceptions of their careers. Another challenge that working nurses experience is feeling respected in the workplace. Public surveys of both physicians and the public indicate nurses are highly respected; however, "respect" means different things to different nurses. Consider the perspective and culture around utilization of nursing resources in any organization you wish to work for. The methods by which they manage nursing resources will give you great insight into their nursing culture and philosophy. Effective communication, collaboration, problem-solving, and teamwork are essential to providing respectful relationships.

Nursing is a great career for men and women who wish to have long-term job security and for those who do well in science courses. There are real positive changes in the RN workforce over the past decade, according to Peter Buerhaus, RN, PhD, FAAN, who has conducted several national nurse surveys: "The increases in work satisfaction and satisfaction with nursing represent . . . positive change in the RN workforce. . . .

We should continue to make improvements in the workplace, improve quality of care and improve relationships with physicians and managers" (Steefel, 2005).

The Nursing Shortage

There have been lots of articles published in both nursing journals and public newspapers across the country about the worldwide nursing shortage. There are really only a few major reasons for this shortage, even though there are many specific intraprofessional issues that have fed into the shortage.

First and foremost is aging of the nursing workforce. The average age of nurses in the United States is 46 (Buerhaus, 2000). There has also been a declining enrollment in nursing programs over the past decade, as women are able to move into other science-focused roles besides nursing (Buerhaus, 2000). Also, high school counselors tend not to recommend nursing to males or to female students interested in the sciences. However, the enrollment trend has reversed within the past two to three years because of increased public awareness of the shortage. Nursing schools now often have waiting lists. Nursing schools in many states do not have the capacity to educate and train nurses as fast as is needed.

The economic climate also allows folks who might consider nursing to choose other careers with higher pay and less stress. The salary structures in many healthcare facilities keep experienced registered nurses at lower salaries compared to other industries. A decreasing emphasis on retention of working nurses by many hospitals has caused nurses to feel that their concerns about stress and patient safety are not being heard or acted upon. Poorly trained managers or brusque, unkind preceptors often leave staff nurses feeling undervalued and not appreciated. These perceptions affect nurses' loyalty to a facility, and therefore become issues that affect job and career choices.

The American Nurses Association (ANA) has created an agenda for the future of nursing that includes discussion about the shortage. ANA believes that there are actually two shortages—a nursing shortage and a staffing shortage. Together, they are causing the problems we are currently facing throughout the country (ANA, 2002).

The staffing shortage is likely due to increased sicker patients with higher acuity, shorter hospital admissions, rising hospital census, the need for changing skill mixes of RNs to accommodate reengineering clinical care of the 1990s, and is defined as "an insufficient number . . . of RNs . . . to safely care for . . . a specific patient population over a specified period of time" (ANA, 2002). The nursing shortage is defined as "the demand and need for RN services greater than the supply of RNs who are qualified, available and willing to do the work" (ANA, 2002). According to the ANA, the causes for the nursing shortage are more professional career opportunities for men and women; an aging nursing workforce; and the public perception of low nursing wages, difficult working conditions, and lack of career growth (ANA, 2002).

Retention is the significant intersection of these two shortages. Retention involves improving the work environment, retaining the aging nursing workforce, improving the image of nursing, and increasing recruitment efforts (ANA, 2002). It is critical to note that by itself, recruitment is *not* enough to assure an adequate supply of nurses. ANA has created a national initiative to deal with the issues that have galvanized the profession. Whereas a national initiative is crucial to mobilize resources, much of what needs to be done rests with state and federal governments and local communities. Every hospital in the country must focus on both retention and recruitment as future cornerstones of an adequate workforce. Producing enough nurses is *everyone's* responsibility.

There was a time it seemed that nurses who worked in administration and those who worked as educators in schools of nursing were actually in two different professions. Contact was limited, and understanding these two different worlds was not relevant much of the time. The differences between these two nursing specialties are not so clear any more. They have many facets in common, not the least of which is sharing the responsibility and challenge of creating competent nurses to meet the shortage.

Although discussion and dialogue have improved, there is much work to be done together to deal with the ever-dwindling supply of nurses. The dialogue created by the forums on the shortage in the late 1990s has resulted in many innovative partnerships between education and service throughout the country. These partnerships have been effective in expanding the supply pipeline of nurses in a specific geographic area and will continue to have a positive impact. However, no nationwide solutions have been proposed to deal with the biggest challenge of creating more nurses—getting students into existing nursing programs.

The individuals most powerfully positioned to assist in this endeavor—state and university college chancellors—so far have turned away from truly innovative methods to increase nursing enrollment. We have legislation, regulation, and numerous innovative ideas, but few real solutions. The nursing faculties in state-college and university programs all over the country are caught in the middle. Nursing student enrollment is dictated by the number of faculty positions available to teach those students. Nursing school educators cannot create more faculty positions on their own, and they are faced with one- to two-year waiting lists of students for nursing programs.

Where are the college chancellors, administrators, and board members in this dilemma? Many large healthcare systems and hospitals have donated large sums of money to fund faculty positions, skills labs, and student tutoring for nursing schools. The hospital industry and professional healthcare organizations have put up thousands of dollars to fund additional nursing students, but the state colleges and universities continue with business as usual. It seems that hospitals and healthcare systems see the nursing-school enrollment issue as a crisis that deserves financial support, but the college systems do not. I find this mindset to be incredibly frustrating as well as mind-boggling.

As you consider which organizations you wish to work in, it is important that you have a good understanding of the organization's progress in dealing with the shortage of registered nurses. It is also critical that they can define action steps to you that they are taking within the organization to manage the precious nursing resources currently employed there.

The current information about the nursing shortage cites these positive signs about those entering and working in the nursing profession. Peter Buerhaus, PhD, RN, and his colleagues found that RN employment has increased and improved since 2001. Over 200,000 RNs have entered the workforce since 2001. Young RNs between ages 21 and 24 increased by 87,000 in 2003, as opposed to second-career students. The average employment growth for nurses of ages 50 to 64 increased 20% between 2001 and 2003. The average employment of foreign-born nurses increased 12.5% between 2001 and 2003. Many facilities are focusing on foreign-born nurses who already live in the United States because the immigration process has become very costly and time-consuming. Nursing wages have increased, and RNs in hospital settings earned more than those outside hospitals (Buerhaus, 2000).

Entering Nursing as a Second Career

Almost half of the students in nursing programs are entering nursing school after completing an education and working in another field (Buerhaus, 2000). Some of these individuals have experienced a layoff or reduction in force in their primary profession. Many choose nursing because they are unhappy in their primary career choice.

If you are choosing nursing as a second career, be sure to evaluate nursing programs specifically geared for individuals who already have a degree or training in another field. There are programs, usually accelerated, that will provide both nursing courses and general-education prerequisites at the same time.

Entry-level MSN programs are particularly popular with second-career RNs. Individuals who already have a bachelor's degree in another field do not want to start over. This desire to pursue nursing without a bachelor's degree in the field is a common

For Your Toolkit

If you are choosing nursing as a second career, be sure to evaluate nursing programs specifically geared for individuals who already have a degree or training in another field.

request and schools are adapting quickly. There are about 50 entry-level MSN programs in the nation, with 20 more in the planning stages (Stringer, 2005). It doesn't make sense to drive second-career nurses into AD (associate degree) programs when they could enter a compressed BSN and regular MSN program instead. Most of these programs take three years to complete. The BSN portion is accelerated and is earned in 12 to 18 months. The master's degree is finished in the following 18 months to 2 years. These programs are rigorous and attract far more applicants than they can accept.

Many entry-level MSN students are motivated to work hard, based on previous baccalaureate course work and their first-career dissatisfaction. Their time in the career world has given them success as well as a degree. They spend a lot of time making the decision to enter nursing, and make mature career decisions because they are older and more experienced (Stringer, 2005). Most students perceive these programs as expensive, but worth it! Information on these types of programs can be found on the Web sites listed here.

Many folks entering nursing after working in another field believe they are at a disadvantage coming into a nursing program. This is not the case. Nursing students with previous work and study experience are very successful. You can take your work experiences and life wisdom from another field into nursing school. Most second-career nursing students need to continue working while attending nursing school. While this is a challenging schedule, it is not impossible. Most nursing programs hold classes two to three days per week, and most healthcare facilities are willing to adjust employee schedules to allow students to attend nursing school.

> **Web sites on nursing schools, accreditation, and scholarships:**
>
> www.nln.org
> www.aacn.nche.edu
> www.discovernursing.com
> www.choosenursing.com
> www.allnursingschools.com
> www.fastweb.com

Men in Nursing

Nursing is becoming better recognized as a successful profession for men. It is interesting that nursing is still considered by many to be a female profession. According to Buerhaus (2003), men now represent 9% of the total nurse labor market. In reality, healers have always come from either gender. Nursing goes back more than 2,000 years, and most of the nurses then were men. The first nurses practiced in ways similar to what we currently consider community health nursing.

The first nursing school was developed in 250 BCE, in India. It was believed that only men were "pure" enough to provide nursing care. In the Byzantine Empire, nursing was considered a separate occupation, only for men. The first documentation of nursing care is in the Bible, with the parable of the Good Samaritan. In that story, a man paid an innkeeper to care for an injured patient. No one thought it odd that a male was to be paid for providing nursing care (Wilson, 1997).

The first hospital was established in 300 CE to provide care for sufferers of the Black Plague. Men were the providers of nursing care. The Benedictine and St. Alexis Orders were the first two religious groups to embrace nursing as a mission. The Alexian Brothers order started its nursing school in the 1300s and still practice nursing today.

There were many famous nurses in the Middle Ages, including Knights Hospitalers and the Knights of St. Lazarus. In the 1800s, during England's Crimean War, men in the military provided all the nursing care. Florence Nightingale was the first person in England recognized as a professional nurse. The first nurses in the United States were acknowledged as such around the time of the Pilgrims, and they were mostly men. It wasn't until the late 1800s that women became the majority of nursing-care providers.

Nursing is a role suited to both sexes. Men in nursing find they can support a family and have much to offer patients because they are men. There are myths surrounding nursing as a "women's profession" that are keeping men from considering a career serving others. With fewer than 10% of nurses licensed in the United States being men, much work must be done to recruit men into this profession, especially men who have served in medical roles in the military. There are now organizations, such as the American Association of Men in Nursing, that focus on recruiting men into the nursing profession.

Selecting a School of Nursing

As the Monster.com healthcare career advisor, and when coaching others, I am asked frequently how to select a nursing school. There are several important factors to consider when selecting a nursing school. First of all, you need to understand the forces working within health care today. There are several driving forces for higher education in nursing. There is increased demand for bachelor's-prepared and advanced-practice master's-prepared nurses. The demand for nurses will increase within the next two decades and the supply will continue to shrink as the Baby Boomers age.

There are numerous reports, such as those from the Pew Commission, ARISTA II, Seventh Report to Congress, Department of Health and Human Services, Department of Labor, and the California Strategic Planning Commission for Nursing, that link a bachelor's degree education level to future needs for nurses. As healthcare delivery continues to shift to outpatient and community sites, differentiating RNs prepared at the associate-level degree from those at the baccalaureate and master's level will increase. Job opportunities and salaries will rise higher and faster for BSN- and MSN-prepared nurses.

Whether these predictions will come true is disputed by some experts in nursing and health care. Whether they are fair to nurses without a baccalaureate degree is up for debate. Fair or not, I believe these trends are real, and nurses need to prepare for them now by carefully considering whether to prepare for nursing in a bachelor's degree program.

For Your Toolkit

If you are choosing nursing as a second career, be sure to evaluate nursing programs specifically geared for individuals who already have a degree or training in another field.

There are many considerations when you are contemplating entering or returning to school, especially if you are considering nursing as a second career. Among the most obvious are your personal values and a passion for the nursing profession, which become the framework for turning a personal dream into an achievable goal by attending nursing school. You will have good employment options, especially if you enter a baccalaureate program, and you will have a chance to enjoy lifelong learning. You will also likely experience changes in your lifestyle and financial status that will affect your family and friends once you decide to enter nursing school. You will spend long hours studying and may need to reduce your work hours to part time to keep up with school demands.

Licensed Practical/Vocational Nurse or Registered Nurse?

The first question to answer is whether you want to be a licensed practical (vocational) nurse (LPN/LVN) or a registered nurse (RN). LPNs and LVNs are called different things in different parts of the United States. LPN/LVNs are considered technical nurses and have 12 to 18 months of training. They are licensed, but must perform many duties under the direct supervision of a professional RN. There are also some nursing tasks that LPN/LVNs are not allowed to perform.

The disallowed tasks vary by state but include patient assessment, patient education, and evaluation of care. LPN/LVNs can perform data collection, reinforce a patient education plan developed by the RN, and provide data from which the RN can evaluate care. LPN/LVNs can work in hospitals, but most find employment in long-term care facilities, clinics, and physician offices. Salaries and job options for LPN/LVNs are limited when compared to RNs. Even with the acute shortage of RNs, LPN/LVNs are not used in hospitals as much as RNs are.

I have worked with many excellent LPN/LVNs in my career. However, the reality is that most of the educational programs, job options, and scholarships are focused on RNs. If you are considering becoming a nurse, enter an RN program. You will earn more and have more options than if you obtain an LPN/LVN license.

If you *are* currently an LPN/LVN, you can usually enter most RN programs at the end of the first year. Contact your local nursing schools to determine their requirements for admitting LPN/LVNs. Some states have specific RN-program entrance requirements for LPN/LVNs. Many healthcare systems, such as Kaiser Permanente, encourage and will pay for LPN/LVNs to complete an RN program while working at their facility.

For Your Toolkit

If you are considering becoming a nurse, enter an RN program. You will earn more and have more options than if you obtain an LPN/LVN license.

When you decide on an RN program, you must determine whether you wish to obtain an Associate Degree in Nursing (ADN) or a Bachelor of Science in Nursing (BSN). An ADN program takes about two years to complete. However, most students entering nursing do not have all the required science courses to enter the nursing program. Therefore, it usually takes another 12 to 18 months to complete the prerequisite science courses. This makes the completion time of an ADN program closer to three and a half years after admission. Most ADN programs require prerequisite courses in math, English, history or sociology, microbiology or biology, chemistry, anatomy, and physiology. Some programs also require an additional fine arts or communication arts course.

ADN programs are offered primarily at community colleges. BSN programs are offered at both private and state colleges and universities. It takes four years to complete a BSN program, including prerequisites. If there is any possible way for you to complete a BSN program, it will be worth the extra time and money. The time spent in an ADN and BSN program is almost the same when you consider the time spent getting prerequisite courses completed for the ADN program. You will have more job options and a higher salary when you graduate. You will only need 18 to 24 months more to complete a master's degree. You are then eligible for many more nursing positions, including management, once you have some professional nursing experience under your belt.

Use the Web sites and resources listed at the end of the book to learn more about nursing schools in your area. There are programs specifically geared to those who are entering nursing as a second career. These programs have been developed in the past several years and are expanding as the demand for them increases.

Financing Your Nursing Education

You also need to determine how to pay for nursing school. There are a number of ways to pay for your education. Look into financial aid, forgivable loans, tuition reimbursement, and scholarships. Federal Student Aid (FAFSA) is available to all qualifying students, including part-time and community-college students. This money is available whether you go to a community college or to a private university. Grants and scholarships are money awards that do not need to be paid back. They are also called "gift aid" or "free money." Grants and scholarships can be based on financial need, grades, or special talents. Churches, professional associations, cultural groups, and hospitals often give local scholarships. Local scholarships are the easiest kind of financial support to obtain. These scholarships do not appear on national Web sites. Check with your high school or college counselor for information on what is available in your region. You may have a much better chance locally than you do for national scholarships, because local scholarships often receive only a few dozen applicants, and the size of your competition group is much smaller.

Apply for every scholarship you can find. It takes time to complete the paperwork, but some scholarship organizations can't find people to give their money to! Even if it doesn't seem worth the time to apply for a small scholarship, do it anyway. Those combined small scholarships have a way of adding up to big dollars.

Also, be alert to potential scams or fraudulent scholarship information. Some nursing Web sites, such as ChooseNursing.com, warn students about scholarship scams. The Federal Trade Commission cautions parents and students to look and listen for statements that sound too good to be true. If you think you have been a victim of a scholarship scam, contact your high school or college counselor and report it. Bring all your materials and letters to your guidance office or a person in a local college's financial aid office for advice.

If you borrow money to pay for your education, you must pay back your loan once you finish school. The interest on the loan is usually low. Some loans are forgiven if you work in certain underserved areas like county hospitals in low-income communities. Many community hospitals now provide forgivable loans for employees who sign an agreement to work a certain amount of time after graduation. The usual agreement is one year of work for every year of paid education. Another option is student employment or work-study. These are programs that provide money that students work for as part of their financial aid. An example would be working 10–15 hours a week in the college library or health center (ChooseNursing.com, 2004).

Evaluating Nursing Programs

1. Be sure to select an accredited nursing program. In most nursing programs, state licensure is required to operate, and national accreditation is voluntary. Community colleges are less likely to seek national accreditation, but baccalaureate programs are almost always nationally accredited because graduate programs often require graduation from an NLNAC or CCNE accredited program for admission. Nearly 80% of university nursing programs are accredited by CCNE, the accrediting arm of the American Association of Colleges of Nursing. NLNAC is the accrediting arm of National League of Nursing.

2. Consider the location of the school. You will likely be driving there at least three days a week for the duration of the program. You will have additional driving to clinical sites, so pick a school that uses hospitals in the local vicinity. Ask about clinical-site availability. One of the major challenges for nursing schools is finding enough clinical-experience sites for students.

3. Ask about faculty. Are all the positions filled? How many retirements are planned within the time you plan to attend? Find out about the academic ranking of the school by contacting the board of nursing in your state. They keep data on NCLEX or state nursing licensure pass rates by school. You want to attend a school with a pass rate of 80% or better.

4. Assess the prestige of the school and stature of the program in the community. This will give you an idea of the stability of the program, its commitment, and funding for the future. Be wary of online or distance programs that promise you can become a nurse without any clinical rotations. You can't become a nurse in any state without doing clinical rotations in a hospital, as well as in other health facilities. If a nursing program sounds too good to be true, it probably is.

5. Ask about the flexibility of the program. Do they offer full-time day classes only? How many days per week must you be on campus? Are there weekend or evening classes? Is the schedule of classes and clinical hours such that you can continue to work full or part time if you have a family to support? Do they use off-site distance learning, video conferencing, online, CD-ROM, or other learning modalities?

6. Evaluate the curriculum. The length of the program will be based on whether you choose an ADN or BSN program. The curricula, at a minimum, should include interdisciplinary practice experiences, have a primary or community-care focus,

and include components on health promotion and prevention, critical thinking, decision-making, supervising the work of others, information technology, health-care financing and policy, and cultural diversity.

7. Ask about tutoring and skills assistance to ensure successful completion of the program. Most nursing schools have skills lab assistants to help you learn clinical skills and tutors who will provide assistance with academic classes. The biggest challenge in nursing school is reading the required material. You will need college-level reading ability, so if reading is difficult for you, consider taking additional reading courses to improve your chances for success.

You will need to evaluate the entire program in each school you consider on the basis of your previous learning needs and experience, any clinical experience, and the need to be mentored and tutored. Be sure you find the best fit for you.

It takes about three to six months to be processed as a nursing school candidate for most schools of nursing, so be sure you check the school application dates and apply early. Sometimes you will need to apply to the college *and* to the school of nursing— two separate applications. Some schools have specific requirements for each program within the school, so be sure you check into that before mailing your application.

Once you are accepted, you will receive written notification and an explanation of what you need to do next. Those steps vary by school and are individualized by campus. It may also be helpful to read one of the student guides currently available for nursing students on how to be successful in nursing school. If you are required to complete CPR certification or other prerequisites prior to entering the program, get them completed early. Most schools of nursing require current certification in CPR as well as certified nurse aide skills. Don't wait until the last minute to complete these prerequisites because doing so may jeopardize your admission.

The topic of how to get through nursing school is an entire book by itself. The most important aspect of getting through school is . . . endurance. You get through it one day at a time. Keys to success when you go to nursing school include keeping your objective in focus, finding a mentor to coach you, and finding a role model to emulate.

Get a commitment upfront from your employer, supervisor, personal support systems, and significant others to support your efforts during the program.

Plan a balance of school, work, self, family, and friends. You can't focus on school to the exclusion of everything else. Be realistic about how much you can work outside while in school. Evaluate the financial ramifications of entering nursing school *before* you start. Remember that good planning, organization, and time management are mandatory for success. Use tuition reimbursement, financial aid, and loans to ease the burden while in school. Become skilled on a computer before you enter the program.

Many nursing students are also primary breadwinners in single-parent families. This means they must work while attending nursing school. Most nursing programs have changed scheduling of classes to accommodate this trend in second-career and older nursing students. If you do work during nursing school, try to balance school, work, and family time. Also, even though it is difficult, carve out some time for yourself that isn't spent studying or doing laundry. You need to recharge yourself in order to care for children, patients, and yourself.

You may want to work as a student worker in the hospital you plan to work in when you complete nursing school. Most state Boards of Nursing have a "student worker" status for nursing students, which allows the students to work to the level of their education and training. There are specific requirements with clear limitations on what student workers can and cannot do. Therefore, even if nursing student workers are not yet licensed as an RN, they can do procedures and administer medications under the direct supervision of a licensed RN preceptor while in their last year of nursing school. Being able to perform additional duties outside the scope of certified nurse aide and patient care techs is a big help to hospitals. This employment status also gives student nurses a chance to learn about the role of the RN from firsthand experience. Most students who work while in school find they can enhance skills, create strong relationships with experienced nurses, and gain valuable experience.

Chapter 2
Life as a New Nurse

Your Interim Permit or Interim License

When you successfully complete and graduate from an accredited nursing program, you must apply for an interim permit or interim license. This permit allows you to work as an interim permittee (IP) or interim licensed (IL) RN. Interim permittee status is only in effect from the time you graduate from nursing school until the time you receive the results of your NCLEX or state board exams. It usually lasts for about three to four months.

Interim permits are issued by your state board of nursing. They usually can be obtained online via board Web sites or by mail. Interim permits allow nursing-school graduates to work as IPs while waiting to take their nursing exams. This means IPs can administer medication, perform procedures, and take physician orders under the direct supervision of a licensed registered nurse. This status lasts only until the state board results are made available. You are then either a registered nurse or no longer an IP. If you need to retake the nursing exams (many nurses do), you can apply for an IP again prior to the next exams. Some states have time limits on when you can sit for an exam after being unsuccessful. Most states allow you to take the exams the next time they are offered.

When you obtain your nursing interim permit, you are a graduate nurse. You are entering the nursing profession as a novice, or someone who has education but little or no experience. This is your opportunity to learn from more experienced nurses.

You can hope that you will work with nurses who are passionate about their profession, kind, and willing to help you be successful.

Your First Nursing Job After Graduation

Many new grads know before they take their state nursing exams where they will be working once they finish school. Most hospitals offer jobs to new graduate nurses as soon as they have finished school. In most states, nurses are able to work with an interim license until they take and pass their state licensing exam. You must market yourself to find that first nursing job. Marketing yourself as a new grad includes standing out from other new grads, using your professional network to find out where the jobs are, looking the part of a nursing professional, and creating a useful resume that will guarantee you an interview.

It is tempting to take the first offer you get as a new grad, but it pays to spend time looking at different facilities before accepting any offers. Don't make a quick decision and accept a position after a first interview. You owe it to yourself and your future to conduct your own research about the facilities where you interview. It is always a good idea to interview in more than one healthcare facility. Even if you are certain you want to work in only one specific location or unit, be sure to do multiple interviews in several facilities, so you can make comparisons.

When you conduct your research, be sure to look at Internet sites for the facility, look up newspaper and journal articles, and review annual reports. Talk to anyone you know who works at a facility where you wish to work. You will learn as much about the facility from those who work there as you will from the individuals who interview you. Your first job sets the stage for the rest of your nursing career. Choose wisely so you will be able to get grounded in your profession right away. Making a poor first job choice may mean you need to leave a facility and start over elsewhere.

For Your Toolkit

Your first job sets the stage for the rest of your nursing career. Choose wisely so you will be able to get grounded in your profession right away.

No matter where you choose to work, be sure you determine what type of orientation and specialty education programs are available for new graduate nurses. Ask specific questions about how long your orientation will be, if you will be assigned a preceptor, and when you will be allowed to care for patients on your own.

If you are not in an orientation program for at least one to two months, you will not be adequately prepared to work as a professional nurse. Being unprepared will lead to increased stress, feelings of inadequacy, and decreased self-esteem and self-confidence. It will also affect your clinical competency. Even if you successfully passed nursing-school courses, graduated with honors, and passed the state nursing exam, you are most likely not ready right away to practice nursing by yourself with no support from experienced staff.

Some facilities offer RN Residencies for new grads. RN Residencies are formal education programs that last from three to six months. Residencies offer formal curricula, designated preceptors and mentors, and structured clinical experiences on the unit where you will work. Trying to function as a new nurse without the benefit of the experience offered in an RN Residency is much like trying to swim races in a pool without having any practice in swimming skills. I believe that RN Residencies should be and will become the new standard for orientation and experiential training of new graduate nurses.

For Your Toolkit

RN Residencies will become the new standard for orientation and training of new graduate nurses.

An exceptional RN Residency program is offered by Versant/Children's Hospital in Los Angeles, California. The outstanding residency developed there will become a model for others across the country. The Versant RN Residency is an innovative, multimodal product that combines an educational process with operational outcomes and management tools. This comprehensive immersion program is designed to help newly graduated registered nurses make the transition from student to competent professional. The many facets of the RN Residency allow facilities to prepare competent, safe, and confident nurses, and simultaneously manage complex operational issues such as recruitment, retention, and nurse self-confidence. The RN Residency program research and evaluation process allows facilities to quantify statistically operational risk of new-grad turnover and degrees of organizational loyalty (Versant, 2005).

The Versant RN Residency has documented its benefits both in elevating the standard of care in the nursing profession and optimizing the financial performance of hospitals. Hospitals all make significant investments in recruitment, training, and retention of RNs but, because of the fragmented approach used, have not achieved the success in turnover reduction that the Versant RN Residency provides. Versant uses a standard core curriculum, combined with a disciplined implementation process and rigorous residency research and evaluation. It is the residency evaluation that provides organizations with analytical results that support proactive monitoring of loyalty rates and potential turnover risks (Versant, 2005). If you have an opportunity to work in a facility that has an RN Residency (especially the Versant model), sign up! It would be a great transition experience, and you would likely stay in that environment for several years.

If a RN Residency program is not available at the facility where you wish to work, ask about formal orientation and precepting options. You definitely want to work at a facility with a formal orientation program. You will have to attend nursing and facility orientation with all new employees. However, once those are completed, you will still need orientation to the role of the professional nurse. Ask the interviewer how that is accomplished in the particular facility. If they cannot present an organized and formalized process or program to you and do not assign you a preceptor for a minimum of three months, reconsider working there.

Many new grads get frustrated and leave nursing within the first year after graduation. This happens because their orientation to professional nursing was poor or nonexistent. It is not reasonable to expect someone right out of nursing school to be competent, safe, and confident with two weeks of hospital orientation and nothing else. Don't sell yourself or your patients short. Insist on formal orientation and an individual preceptor before you accept your first registered nurse position.

Having a Life *and* a Career: Achieving Life Balance

Because your first job sets the tone for your first professional nursing experience, it is critical that you be well prepared for it. In addition to a formal orientation program as discussed previously, you must also find a way to balance your life. Nursing is a stressful profession, so you need some self-care strategies to make the most of your life and your nursing role.

Most important, when you start a new job, remember that you do not have to know everything. It is a myth that healthcare employers expect new nurses to know all there is to know about being a nurse. Even experienced nurses start out as novices when they take on a new role. It is okay to not know things. You are not expected to know everything. Remind yourself of that every day!

Employers do expect nurses to deliver safe and competent care to patients. That is why choosing a job with a formal orientation program or a RN Residency is so important. There is a steep learning curve for all newly hired nurses. How fast you learn is individual and different for each nurse. You are not expected to know everything. Asking for help will not label you as incompetent or a burden. Ask for help *before* you drown. You are not expected to be perfect, but rather to know what you don't know. It is also important for you to ask questions about situations and care practices you are not familiar with. You are responsible for telling your supervisor if you are not trained for or have never performed a specific skill that you are asked to do as a new nurse.

Nursing is a profession where safety and precision are significant. Policies and procedures exist to ensure that nothing is taken for granted and care is provided in the safest way possible. Policies and procedures may seem cumbersome and time-consuming, but they are created as safeguards to protect patients. It is crucial that you ask for and follow facility procedures and policies to avoid errors that may endanger patients, their families, or fellow staff members. The reality check that occurs after you make a mistake that significantly affects a patient outcome is not the way to start your nursing career.

Because you can't know everything, it is important to know where to find the information you need. Cultivate resources and use them. Internet Web sites, policy and procedure manuals, textbooks, "How to be a new grad" booklets, and pocket guides are all useful tools to gather information. Preceptors are often designated for new grads or experienced nurses in a new position. You should request one if you are not assigned one as a new grad. You can consult other nurses besides your preceptor to mentor or coach you. Find an experienced RN that you trust and use him/her as a guide when you are unsure of how to proceed.

For Your Toolkit

Find a nurse you can trust to be your mentor or coach. Use this person as a guide when you are unsure of how to proceed.

It is also a good idea to find someone to answer questions when you move to a new unit or shift. When you switch to the night shift, which most new grads do during their first year, you need advice. It is really helpful to have someone who already works nights tell you how to survive the hours, manage family, find sleeping strategies, and other tips. If you move or float to another unit, find a person who seems approachable and ask how they suggest you begin. Unfortunately, not everyone will be friendly and helpful, but you will find most staff eager to share their experiences and ideas.

Common courtesy and graciousness go a long way when you are new on a job. They are as important to your success as clinical skills. "Please" and "thank you" are not out of style and will make experienced staff more willing to assist you with questions. As Joan Duncan Oliver says, "Kindness is one of the most undervalued commodities . . . " (Hill, 1998). Be pleasant to everyone and try to avoid joining a clique in your new workplace. It is likely that there will be work groups or cliques already formed in your new unit. Be careful about being drawn into one, especially the special-interest groups that are negative or nonproductive.

For Your Toolkit

Common courtesy and graciousness are as important for success as clinical skills.

Try and meet new people every day. Don't be shy in the cafeteria; introduce yourself to staff from other departments. Find out what their role is in your facility. Some facilities even have "welcome" programs. These programs ask that other staff introduce themselves to new staff and explain where they work. This strategy is a great way to meet new people and discover resources in other departments.

Keep in mind that, although it is a great idea to reach out to work with others, you need to maintain healthy boundaries for yourself. As the "newbie" on the unit, you will be asked by other staff to work a weekend, take an extra shift, or to perform other tasks. Don't let other staff take advantage of you. If you wish to work extra, that's great. But if you would rather not, then don't. Remember, it is okay to maintain your boundaries and individuality and to say "no."

You will be learning many new things each day in your first job as a professional nurse. Consider journaling your ideas, problems, solutions, and strategies each day as a way of reflecting on as well as storing information. If you used reflective journaling in nursing school, you are already familiar with the format. You don't need anything fancy to write in or special writing talents. Just write about your shift, thoughts, feelings, and ideas. It is a great stress reducer.

Remember, you have been trained to be a problem-solver and to use critical-thinking skills. Although health care demands precision and specificity, there are also many areas that are unclear, with differences of opinion as well as gray areas. You will find that even the experts disagree on specific procedures and processes for some nursing tasks. You will likely develop your own opinions and ideas once you have some patient-care experience. Focus on critical-thinking strategies and problem-solving skills to stay balanced.

Last but definitely not least, you need to take care of yourself. You cannot care for others effectively without caring for yourself first. This is true while you are caring for patients, raising children, and interacting with family members, spouses, or significant others. You need to identify ways you can disconnect from your work. Do something—yoga, meditation, walking the dog, listening to music, taking baths—whatever it takes to let you unplug and reflect.

Also plan some alone time for yourself. Alone time isn't selfish or being irresponsible. Keep in mind that alone time is doing something for your soul space. Alone time is not going to the grocery store, doing laundry, or commuting to work. Make an appointment with yourself and do something renewing. You deserve some time alone

Turner Stress Assessment Tool©

For the purposes of this test, stress is defined as a mismatch between the demands placed on you and your ability to meet those demands.

Circle the correct response for you. There are no "right" answers!

1. Do you feel stressed at work?   Yes   No

2. Do you feel more stressed at work now than you did three years ago?   Yes   No

3. Do you feel more stressed at work now than you did one year ago?   Yes   No

4. How stressed do you feel right now?   Not at all   Not much   Fairly   Some   Very

5. If you feel stressed, how does this manifest itself? Circle all that apply:

   Physically

   Headaches   Stomach/bowel problems   Chest pain
   Frequent infections   Sleep problems   Weight loss
   Weight gain   Loss of libido

   Psychological

   Moodiness/irritability   Tiredness   Apathy   Depression
   Anxiety   Frustration   Indecision   Boredom
   Feeling guilty   Poor concentration

(continues)

Turner Stress Assessment Tool© (continued)

Behaviorally

Accident-proneness   Alcohol abuse   Drug abuse
Food abuse   Aggressiveness   Relationship difficulties
Absenteeism

6. How do you feel stress in your personal life affects you at work?
    Not at all   A little   Quite a bit   A lot

7. How do you feel stress at work affects your personal life?
    Not at all   A little   Quite a bit   A lot

8. If you feel stressed, what would you say are the major sources of
    your stress?
    Excessive workload   Lack of resources   Staff   Management
    Patients   Personal difficulties   Changes within profession
    Job insecurity   Job transition/new job

9. How do you cope with stress?
    Counseling   Support groups   Recreational activities
    Relaxation   Stress-management techniques
    Talking with friends/significant other   Regular exercise
    Alcohol/drugs/nicotine/food   Missing work   Denial

10. How would you rate your ability to cope with stress?
    Poor   Average   Better than average   Very good

11. How many stress-related sick leave/days have you used in the past
    year?

Turner Healthcare Associates, Inc., © 1994.

without justifying it by multitasking. Dr. Phil McGraw (2005) says that quality alone time must nourish your relationship with yourself. His rule of thumb is, "If you were doing the same activity with your kids, would it nourish your relationship with them?" Watching a movie may be enjoyable, but it doesn't bring you closer to the person you are sitting next to. Since alone time is about building a relationship with yourself, the same is true. Everyone is different. You don't have to sit alone and stare at the walls. Find a way to look inward. Write in a journal. Create a life plan. Create a career plan. Take a walk. Have a massage. Do whatever works for you to focus inwardly and renew yourself.

Nursing is a rewarding profession, but it is stressful and takes energy out of your body and soul. Be sure you refill your "energy pot" and your soul space to keep yourself healthy and able to provide care. Finding private time for yourself will refill your soul and renew your spirit. Remember that being a nurse is more than being competent. It is about being of service. In order to be of service, you must have energy to work with.

Chapter 3
Career Development

Career development means taking total responsibility for your career and your life. Career success is not a matter of luck, nor does it just happen—it requires careful planning and analysis. Moving through a career is often thought to be like climbing a ladder, with different roles at higher and higher levels. In reality, your nursing career is more like a tree, with many branches and limbs on which to gain experience. Every job and role you take allows you to gather more experience, skills, and competencies to put in your career toolkit. The more tools you have in your toolkit, the more marketable you are.

For Your Toolkit

Career success requires careful planning and analysis.

Part of career development includes assessing your educational level. Nursing is a career that embraces lifelong learning. If you have graduated from a hospital diploma program or a community college program, have you continued your professional learning after graduation? How? It is important to include an educational evaluation in your career assessment. It is important to evaluate what other career options you may have or cannot pursue because you have not enhanced your education level.

Going back to school to earn a bachelor's or master's degree is not for everyone. But you owe it to yourself to evaluate what it would mean to your career to do so. You can always decide not to go back to school, but at least you have evaluated what education means to you and your career development. If you do decide to go back to school, that additional learning will never be wasted, no matter what career choices you make.

Manage Your Career

According to Dan Thomas (1994), you must manage your career like a business. Most people do not use good business sense in managing their careers. Over the years, Thomas has observed that the best students and the best managers are not always the most successful in their personal careers. Why? What makes the difference between success and failure in a career? Is it contacts, luck, or plain hard work? All of these components are helpful, but no single factor is the determining cause for success or failure.

Thomas believes there are specific things you can do to enhance the chances of success with your career. The first two are crucial, but few people give them any thought. First, choose the right organization. Most folks don't recognize the obvious: Whenever you have a choice, choose a great organization. Health care is a very successful business. It is a growing industry with many opportunities for nurses. However, not every healthcare organization is a great place to work.

Second, choose the right strategy. This may seem obvious, but many folks don't consider their own career strategies important. Strategies are the decisions you make to position yourself in a complex environment (Thomas, 1994). A complex environment certainly describes the typical healthcare organization! You must make the choice to manage your strategies actively or do nothing and let the environment make decisions for you. Doing nothing is never a good idea. Most people mistakenly believe that if they do a good job, they will be successful. Nothing is further from the truth. To be perceived as being successful, you must market yourself by differentiating your skills so that what you offer is uniquely important to the organization where you work.

For Your Toolkit

Being an indispensable nurse means your skills will always be in demand.

You may be wondering how to do this in a hospital when there are many other nurses doing exactly the same tasks you are. The answer is to become indispensable. It is not difficult to be perceived by your boss and organization as indispensable. It is all about how you position yourself in the organization and how you are perceived. The traits of an indispensable nurse include the ability to:

- demonstrate clinical competence.
- demonstrate leadership skills—planning, coordinating, delegating, supervising the work of others.
- commit and practice lifelong learning, including professional development.
- grasp professional changes in your organization (patient safety focus, increased regulatory and financial requirements).
- be willing to partner with co-workers and your organization to achieve success.
- exercise independence and self-direction.
- be motivated with high energy.
- be objective and nonpartisan toward special-interest mentalities.
- demonstrate integrity.
- demonstrate flexibility and adaptability.
- use good time management.
- be assertive and tenacious.
- have a general understanding of the Joint Commission on Accreditation of Healthcare Organizations (JCAHO) and other regulatory mandates.
- provide positive role-modeling to other staff members.

Turner Healthcare Associates, Inc., ©1998.

The third thing Thomas suggests for career success is to develop the right systems. Patient care processes and systems rely on information. Information is crucial for you to be successful. Having the right information at the right time is very important. Many people measure career success by looking at their past performance. This is only part of the picture. As important as it is to look backward, it is more important to look ahead—as Wayne Gretsky says, "go where the puck is."

To get to "where the puck is," you must evaluate the skills and abilities of the people at your level in the healthcare industry. What are the leaders in your organization and throughout the industry doing to develop themselves and stay ahead of the competition? Read as much as you can and talk to those who know what skills will be required of nurses in the future. Then you will know how to market yourself.

For Your Toolkit

Assess your career at regular intervals and actively plan your next steps.

Turner Indispensable Nurse Assessment Tool©

Are you in a position of being indispensable to your boss or unit? Take this assessment to see how indispensable you are. The more "yes" answers you have, the more indispensable you are!

1. Are you clinically competent?

2. Do you have a general understanding of JCAHO accreditation and requirements?

3. Do you have a general understanding of managed-care issues that affect your geographic area?

4. Do you have a general understanding of budget and cost issues that affect your facility?

5. Are you willing to be a partner with your institution, not just an employee?

6. Do you have decision-making skills?

7. Are you self-directed, not always expecting to be told what to do?

8. Do you have integrity?

9. Do you have an objective perspective?

10. Do you act like a victim?

(continues)

Turner Indispensable Nurse Assessment Tool© (continued)

11. Do you have a strong work ethic? (Not a workaholic.)

12. Do you have a high energy level?

13. Do you have effective time-management skills?

14. Do you have a strong, positive self-image?

15. Do you have effective interpersonal skills?

16. Are you flexible?

17. Are you excited, not threatened, by change?

18. Can you deal with change and get mobilized, even if you are afraid?

19. Are you adaptable?

20. Are you assertive?

21. Are you tenacious?

22. Do you have personal ambition and drive?

23. Are you self-motivated and a self-starter?

Turner Healthcare Associates, Inc., ©1998.

Fourth, you must design the right career support structure. Individuals need a support structure for career management. This structure consists of mentors, colleagues, coaches and subordinates to help them achieve their objectives. Colleagues and subordinates who can cooperate with you and have complementary skills can be sources for future success (Thomas, 1994). You can use mentors in your support structure in an active way or passive way. You will likely need both types of mentors in nursing. (See Chapter 7 on mentors/coaches.) Remember that simply doing a good job does not guarantee success. You must create your own success.

> **To improve the chance of success in your career:**
>
> - choose a great organization to work for.
> - use effective strategies for positioning yourself in the workplace.
> - make yourself indispensable, innovative, and unique to your organization.
> - create effective information loops and support structure.
> - enhance all types of communication skills.
> - think outside the box about your job and your career.

Create a Plan

As you gain experience as a professional nurse, you will need to use a career development plan. This plan will have several stages. I created the Turner Career Development Model© while working on my dissertation. You need to think critically about your career path at regular intervals during your life. I evaluate my situation on my birthday every year. Start by doing an assessment. You can use the Turner Career Self Assessment Tool© or create your own method. Look at what you are doing and how it is working for you. Complete the assessment and then evaluate your situation.

- What are you missing in job skills?
- Are you passionate about your work?
- Do you want to work as a manager?

Once you complete an assessment, then you can create a plan. The Turner Career Development Tool© and Turner Career Planning Process© will assist you in drafting a personal plan for yourself. You must determine how you will get yourself through the transition process that is generated when you make life changes. Take a look at the Turner Transition Model© (Figure 8-1) and Chapter 8 on workplace transition for more information on transition and change.

Turner Career Self Assessment Tool©

1. The tasks and components I like most about my present job are:

2. The tasks and components I like least about my present job are:

3. The tasks I excel at in my present job are:

4. The tasks I struggle with in my present job are:

5. My educational goals are:

6. My lifelong learning goals are:

7. My short-term (within one year) goal(s) is (are): By the year 20__, I will have:

8. The steps I need to take to achieve this short-term goal are:

9. My long-term (two to three years) goal(s) is (are): By the year 20__, I will have:

10. The steps I need to take to achieve this long-term goal are:

11. Jobs outside the acute-care hospital that interest me are:

12. Areas of cross training or specialization within the hospital that interest me are:

13. The resources I need to achieve my short-term and long-term goals are:

Turner Healthcare Associates, Inc., ©1994.

Turner Career Development Tool©

1. What are you doing now? Describe your work and role.

2. What do you want and need in a job and role? (list points from the self-assessment tool)

3. Gather information about the roles you like: what do you know about these roles? What do you like about them? What else can you find out? Where? When?

4. Target one or two roles to aim for: What is it? Where is it done? Who do you know that you could job-shadow in this role?

5. Decide which one role you actually want to do. If you had to make a decision today, what would you choose? Why?

6. List and explain four strategies to achieve the role you chose in the previous question.

7. To implement your strategies you would have to do what? How? When? Where?

8. Is furthering your professional education important to you? Why or why not?

9. If you want to further your professional education, what will you do? When? How?

10. Decide on a method for you to continue your ongoing career development and management. What will the method include? When will you do it?

11. How will you know you are successful at achieving your goal(s)? List your criteria for success.

12. What will you do to reward yourself for your success? When?

Turner Healthcare Associates, Inc., ©1994.

Turner Career Planning Process©

1. Where do you want to be in three to five years?

2. What do you want and like in a job?

3. Gather information about the roles you like. List them.

4. Target one or two roles to aim for. List them.

5. Decide on one role to do. List it.

6. Develop five strategies to achieve that role (school, certification, job-shadowing).

7. Implement your five strategies, one at a time.

8. Evaluate your outcomes and continue your ongoing career management.

Turner Healthcare Associates, Inc., ©1994.

Last, but not least, evaluate what you have accomplished. Does this sound familiar? (See Figure 3-1.)

Assessment → Plan → Manage transition → Evaluate

Yes, it is similar to the nursing process you learned in nursing school!

When we talk with our friends and colleagues about their personal lives and dilemmas, we are often able to see the issues very clearly, even when they cannot. Because we are not emotionally involved in their situation, it makes it easier to sort out their critical issues and determine the best way for them to proceed to solve the problem.

That critical-thinking process we use with our friends is the same one we need to apply to our own career evaluation. It is always harder to evaluate your own issues, so you may want some help doing this.

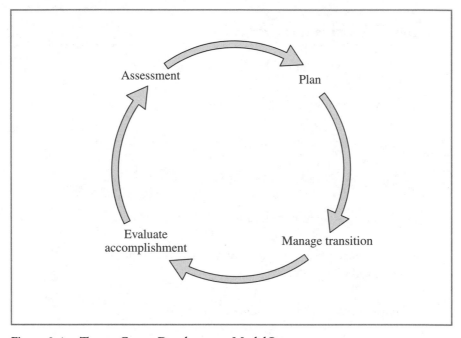

Assessment

Plan

Manage transition

Evaluate
accomplishment

Figure 3-1   Turner Career Development Model©

Career development starts with an assessment of where you are and then deter-mining where you want to be. In addition to using the Turner Career Self Assessment© to plan your personal transition and revitalization, you will also want to create your own plan for the future. To do that, you must implement a career strategy based on critical thinking. It is okay to have more questions than answers.

To get started, make your planning and managing multifaceted. Be sure to include both your life responsibilities and your career in your assessment. You may want to set new goals for yourself and with your manager as you move through the assessment process. You can choose experts to assist you at different aspects of your career.

Assess your educational level and future educational needs and update your resume annually. Create personal one-year and five-year plans for your career. Identify steps and strategies to implement your career plan. Evaluate what you enjoy and are good at doing. Assess why you love your work. It is important to determine early on if you are going to work at a profession you love, or you are just going to a job.

Nurses must be active in their own career development. Many nurses simply move from job to job without considering long-term strategies or career goals. This can lead to stagnation and burnout. Before you begin, take stock of where you are in your pre-sent job. Are you doing your best? Are you enthusiastic? Burned out? Bored? There are numerous books on how to evaluate your career, but the one I like best is the

Graduate Handbook of Job Searching Techniques (Stern, 1990). I have adapted the process described in that book for my Turner Career Development Tool©.

Start by evaluating your present role. Taking stock of where you are is the most important step of your career planning process. To avoid making choices blindly, you must find out where you are, what you have to offer, and how you fit into the big—and rapidly changing—healthcare industry. Read. Listen. Watch. Learn. Find out as much as you can about the national and local trends in health care. This will tell you what the future opportunities will be. The more insight you have, the better equipped you will be to handle changes in your career.

If Not Now, When?

Some other career development tips include:

- Know who to call—trusted friend or mentor.
- Think out of the box.
- Reach for the stars—anything goes.
- Use the assessment tool to create short- and long-term goals.
- Evaluate income needs versus personal satisfaction.
- Be a risk-taker.
- Consider getting more education.
- Believe you can do whatever you need to be successful.

It is important to design a future for yourself that is a good fit for you and where you are at different stages of life. In their 20s and 30s, most folks have big dreams and make long-range plans. Once you hit your 40s, the ideas change to what makes you happy *now*. It is easy to get caught in the assumption that we are somehow exempt from the passing of time.

We always assume that we can do all the things we dream of doing. We just don't have time to do them now. We think that our life will automatically get better, and that some time in the distant future we will be nicer and finally do things like lose 40 pounds, learn to play the 12-string guitar, and write in a journal.

When you are living the overwhelming grind of working *toward* your future, you end up thinking that you can always do your wish list someday. Suddenly someday is *now*. When you look at where you are going, the future needs to fit who you are becoming. If you are young, realize that your future will change as you age and you will be making this assessment again.

The future when you are age 40 is not the same as when you were younger. Besides financial planning (a *must!*) for your older years, you must also imagine a future from where you are. You need to take an honest look at your life and figure out what future fits where you are now. You need to start the process of creating a future that fits the person you are becoming—not one that fits who you have been. As

Ronna Lichtenberg (2005) suggests, you can write a working scenario and a not-working scenario. Describe it in great detail—who is there, what kind of work or activities you are doing, what you are wearing. Create two scenarios. Consider the best possible future and your worst possible future. Write down the scenario, and then put it away. Give yourself at least a week, and then find time to review both your best- and worst-future versions. Identify with what feels like a big deal to you in both scenarios. Find the clues for what you really want to have in your future that is a change from how you are living your life now (Lichtenberg, 2005).

Once you know this, you can create your action plan. Start with one thing you can do that will take you toward the future you want to have. Your future doesn't have to be in black-and-white answers. It can have "maybes" also. Maybe you can try something different. Maybe you can change jobs. Doing this exercise will help remind you that you are here, now, and that your old future may not fit anymore. You will discover that you are still a work in progress, and that is a good thing.

After you have written your best- and worst-future scenarios, evaluate what they look like. Consider your present job. What do you like? Dislike? What are you good at? Not so good at? Think about what makes you happy in your work. Be honest. Next, think about what you would like and not like in a job. Travel? Management responsibility? Flexible scheduling? Children? Healthy people? Old people? Think about all the issues and be open-minded. Thinking "outside the box" gives you more ways to put together something that will work just right for your life.

Gather information about roles you like. Look on the Web, at advertisements in nursing journals, and talk to colleagues about what their jobs entail. Once you have lots of information, you can choose one or two roles that you want to pursue. Find out all you can about these roles. Make sure they fit well with your professional goals and your personal life. Decide on a role to pursue, and find out about educational requirements, salary, training requirements, and job availability. Consider job-shadowing for a day with someone already in the role you are considering.

Next, you need to plan your strategies. Talk with your current supervisor about your plans. Chances are s/he will support you. Investigate when you can attend school, change your schedule, or rearrange child care to pursue your interest. Make sure you consider all the possibilities. Be flexible in your approach and also make a backup plan for each strategy.

Once you have planned your strategies, you need to implement them. This is easier said than done. You actually have to *do* things—not just talk or read about them. This is where to put your energy into moving forward with your plan. Make sure your supervisor, co-workers, and significant others know you are working toward a professional goal and will need their support and understanding. Most of the time you will find everyone to be supportive. Don't forget to include arrangements for child care during class time, time for class reading, or time to write papers when you are implementing your plan.

More career development tips:

- Work at your own level of professional development.
- Evaluate your own clinical performance.
- Direct your own professional and career growth.
- Pursue your own professional interests and specialties.
- Ask for objective, competency-based performance evaluations focused on the nursing process and on leadership skills.
- Decide whether you want to work toward developing your expertise or preparing for future roles.
- Decide whether more education will enhance your role performance.
- Complete job self-assessment/stress assessment/skills inventories.
- Explore roles that interest you.
- Gather information about the roles that interest you (the education, training, and skills required).
- Target the roles that most interest you.
- Make a decision about the role you will pursue first.
- Strategize about how you will achieve that role.
- Implement your strategy.
- Reward yourself for your success.
- Manage your career regularly and no less than annually (on your birthday or another day each year).

Continue your career management throughout your professional life. Pick a date and assess where you are annually. I usually use my birthday and determine whether I like where I am professionally and what I want to do differently. To do this on an ongoing basis, you must acknowledge your own needs and changing life issues. If you have small children, what you can tolerate professionally is different from when your children are fully grown.

As with other life assessments, be sure you also consider what you cannot do and what you are not. This sounds odd, but you need to be honest about what you cannot do, so you don't set yourself up to get into a job situation where you apply that particular skill all the time. In my case, I would never want a job or role that requires budgeting and financial skills. I can read and manage budgets, but I don't want to spend my time crunching numbers. I am not good at math, and therefore need to include that fact in my career planning. I also get bored easily. I need changing activities to stay passionate about my work. Knowing your limitations is as important as knowing your strengths!

Identify what you need to deal with those limitations. In my case, it means using a really good calculator all the time and having resource people with financial skills.

As you continue to manage your career, be sure you assess where you want to be in the future as well as right now. What do you want to do in two years? In five? What is your personal mission statement? Use the Turner Career Self Assessment Tool© to create your own personal career plan. Understanding these things about yourself is crucial to accurate career planning. Talk to your mentors regularly but no less than once a year. Reward yourself for actually implementing your career plan as well as for successes. It is easy to get bogged down in the details of what you are currently doing. Don't forget what your long-term and future goals are.

Resumes

Having a winning (not just acceptable) resume is the beginning of finding your first job. When human-resource recruiters receive hundreds of resumes a day, their best strategy to narrow down the "keepers" is through the process of elimination. Your resume becomes the only tool to let recruiters know why you would be the right person for the job. You need to create a useful resume.

There are many books available on how to create a resume. You can purchase one, consult online experts at locations like Monster.com, or hire someone to create a resume for you. No matter how you choose to create your resume, here are the most crucial things to remember.

A resume *must* be free of spelling errors, typos, and poor grammar. Always include a cover letter that speaks specifically to the job you are applying for. Use appropriate and professional formatting. Make the resume no longer than two pages. Use bullet points, not long paragraphs. When listing experience versus education, list the heading first where you have spent the most time recently. Be sure you have a resume that explains what your accomplishments are and how you achieved them, not just a listing of job descriptions or tasks. Make sure your hiring dates and employer contact information is accurate and complete. Do not list personal information that is irrelevant to the job you are applying for. Your height, weight, marital status, GPA, and other personal information do not belong in a professional resume. List your previous employment in reverse chronological order. Explain any gaps in your employment in the cover letter, not in the resume. Be honest about your education, titles, training, and previous salary.

When you write a cover letter, include the date, your name, and contact information. List a contact person's name, title, and address. Take the time to find this out, so that you can send a personally addressed cover letter. Add an appropriate salutation. Stay away from "Dear Sir/Madam"—too impersonal. Express your interest in a position or in working at that facility. List the qualifications, experience, and education that makes you the right candidate for the job.

Identify and address any red flags in your resume. If you have gaps in work history or have relocated or left a job, address those issues briefly in your cover letter. Make a philosophical statement about what you bring to the job you are interested in or why you became a nurse. State an action that identifies what you will do next, for example, call next week. Be proactive about getting an interview and call the facility to set one up, unless it is specifically stated that the facility does not want to receive calls.

Interviews

Your mother was right. First impressions really do matter. As has often been said, you never get a second chance to make a first impression. First impressions in job interviews usually make or break the rest of the process. Nursing is a job-seeker's paradise. Even so, nurses should not assume that jobs are always available, or that they "landed the job" after a pleasant interview. Believing that the job is automatically yours because of the large number of vacant positions is risky. Landing a job requires more than just showing up. Interview techniques and expectations have evolved, and the strategies you used 20 years ago won't work anymore. Preparation for an interview is now the most important thing you can do to be successful.

For Your Toolkit

First impressions in job interviews make or break the rest of the process.

Most healthcare interviews now include questions based on a behavioral model. These kinds of questions cannot be answered with a simple "yes" or "no." Behavioral questions are designed to glean specific explanations of scenarios from interviewees and how they would react to a given situation. How applicants answer the questions is as important as what they say. These types of questions are designed to get an interviewee to describe a circumstance that has happened in their past work environment and how they dealt with it. The idea behind these types of questions is that the best predictor of future behavior is past behavior. Be sure to evaluate scenarios in your career that you can address. Those situations that involve conflict resolution, impressive communication strategies, or major contributions are the ones to mention during the interview.

Don't forget to do your homework. Remember, you are interviewing the facility as much as they are interviewing you. You need to research the institution to learn about any specialty areas, the care philosophy, and any specifics about the unit or area you are interviewing for. Arriving prepared for an interview sends the message that you are interested in the facility as much as they are interested in you.

There are several generations active in professional nursing. As Jennifer Hermann, director of workplace planning at UCSF Medical Center, says, "That is a huge age range for ideas, attitudes, and expectations." Many people doing interviews are in their 40s and 50s. They may have very different perceptions of work-related issues than a new grad under age 30. Remember to pay attention to how you are dressed and how you conduct yourself. This will minimize chances for miscommunication. Hermann believes that taking a formal approach when being interviewed by someone like this can show respect for their view of the profession (Cowles, 2005).

Doing Your Interview Homework: Preparing for the Interview

Be sure you can answer the following questions* before going to an interview:

- Will I be effective, with my skills/abilities, working for this employer?
- Are there jobs available in roles I am interested in and qualified for?
- How does this employer treat employees?
- Is this employer financially stable?
- What are the opportunities for advancement? For women?
- How does this organization rank within the healthcare industry?
- What are the services offered by this organization?
- Does this organization have problems that I can use my skills to help solve?
- How do employees who work in this organization feel about their jobs?
- What is the turnover of employees in this organization?
- How does this organization communicate with employees? Externally?
- Does this organization encourage professional development and advancement? Provide scholarships or tuition reimbursement?
- What kind of management style does the person have to whom I would report? Does it blend with my personality and professional characteristics?
- Do I know what the job description requirements/tasks are?

*Adapted from *Nurses Guide to Managed Care*, 1996.

How to Create a Successful Interview

Preparing in advance can help lower your stress level and improve your performance during the process. Research the company to learn as much as you can and make sure it is the right environment for you. Read the facility's mission statement and determine its core values, where its focus is, and some recent successes or achievements. Use and speak about the researched information to demonstrate your knowledge and interest during the interview. Rehearse the interview. Practice your facial expressions, eye contact, handshake, and body language. Practice answering likely interview questions so you don't stumble over the wording.

When planning your schedule, allow at least two hours for the interview. In some cases, you'll actually need an entire day. Professionals dress professionally: Men usually wear ties, dress shoes, and a suit or sportscoat and dress slacks. Women wear blue or black suits, hosiery, and dress shoes. Check yourself in a full-length mirror, front *and* back, before you leave your residence. Avoid displaying anything that may take attention away from your skills and qualifications—trendy fashions, tattoos, nose rings, intense makeup, etc. Arrive at the interview a few minutes early. Always make sure you allow extra time if you are unfamiliar with the location.

Be polite. Show respect to everyone you meet, no matter whether it's the boss, the receptionist, or a prospective co-worker. Shake hands firmly and make eye contact with the interviewer. Know what questions you should answer and what questions are illegal (age, marital status, children, race, religion, sexual preferences, or personal habits). Focus your comments on what you can offer the facility to solve its problems.

Be familiar with your work history and skills. Explain gaps in employment and why you left past jobs. Frame these comments in a positive way. Try and recall specific work situations or scenarios when answering questions. Bring a resume with you. Even if the interviewer has a copy, another can be useful for you to reference as you answer questions.

Gather information and bring it with you: phone numbers, addresses of past employers, employment dates, etc. Bring your license and certifications and specialty training cards (e.g., ACLS). Do not write "see resume" on the application form. Bring a neatly typed list of professional references. Include the relationship of the reference to you and the best way to reach that person. Be sure to contact each person you list as a reference *before* you give the list to an interviewer so your references will not be surprised or uncomfortable about getting a call from a facility.

Think of yourself as a product with features and benefits you want to sell and gear your answers accordingly. Focus on what the interviewer really wants to know. Identify what you are good at task wise—not necessarily the same as "strengths." How will your features benefit this employer? Nurses definitely need good people skills. However, another prerequisite of the job is a measure of technical literacy. Be confident about your skills and explain how your experiences and interests are a match for the position.

Be comfortable talking about yourself. Confidence and enthusiasm are critical characteristics of an interview. Prepare three to five questions to ask the interviewer. Asking insightful questions sets you apart from other applicants. Questions demonstrate that you've done your homework about the company and that you are as interested in finding out how you'll fit in and achieve your career goals as they are in learning whether you're the right person for the job. Ask specific questions about the position: To whom will you report? What are the job expectations? How do they manage people? What is the greatest challenge in the job?

Never ask about salary, number of vacation weeks, or other benefits during a job interview. The time to talk about money and benefits is after the employer has offered you the job.

Follow up with a thank-you letter to the interviewer or a phone call to communicate your interest in the position and to answer any additional questions. In your letter, be sure you address that:

- you heard what specifics the interviewer mentioned about the role.
- you are excited about the job, can do the job, and want the job.
- you have excellent communication skills and will mesh well with the organization.
- you can clear up any confusion, negative impressions, or provide clarifications.

Most recruiters agree that the person who gets the job is not always the best qualified, but the one who knows how to prepare and conduct the best interview. Always keep in mind that basic interview protocols never go out of style. A formal interview approach, professional business attire, and a personal, handwritten thank-you note to follow up are always appropriate and will put you above other job-seekers. Everything you do to obtain a new position, including written communication and how you dress, needs to show that you are highly professional. Remember that the small things can make a really big difference.

Working with a Recruiter*

Many hard-to-find, middle-management and senior executive positions are filled by corporate recruiters. This means that the facility hires a recruiter to find and screen qualified job candidates. A recruiter's job is to provide a pool of qualified candidates for open positions and to help the hiring manager choose the most qualified candidate from that pool to fill the job. There are several types of recruiters and it helps to know the difference. In all but the rarest cases, recruiters represent the hiring entity, not the candidate.

Agency recruiters: Agency recruiters can work independently, be associated with a small "boutique" firm that focuses on a particular industry, or be part of a large firm. Agency recruiters can fill either full-time or temporary positions, but their compensa-

*The author wishes to acknowledge and thank the recruiters who assisted her with developing this chapter. Patricia Nygren and Sutzi McGovern provided invaluable information and insight.

tion always comes as the direct result of filling a position for a client company. If it's a temp position, the agency gets a mark-up over the hourly rate to cover statutory taxes, any benefits offered and paid for by the client company, and the agency's profit margin. If it's a full-time regular position, then compensation usually comes in one of two ways—contingency placement or retained search.

With a *contingency placement*, the agency is paid only when a candidate is hired (and often completes a probationary period). A client company might ask multiple agencies to work on one search and then hire the best candidate. Agencies will work on contingency positions if and only if they think they have a good chance of filling the position in a short amount of time, otherwise the effort exceeds the rewards. Contingency searches are usually done when there is a large candidate pool for one position.

On a *retained search*, the agency is paid a fee to fill a position, and they work on the search until the position is filled. The fee is generally paid in installments— usually one third up front, one third upon presentation of three qualified candidates, and one third upon candidate placement. The agency is also usually reimbursed for all of their expenses, including travel to interview candidates. Retained searches are usually chosen for professional-level positions only, and almost always at the management and executive levels.

Executive recruiters: Executive search firms (technically agencies, but they don't like to be called that!) specialize in filling positions at the management and executive levels. They rarely get involved with temp work or temp positions. Almost all of their work is handled on a retained-search basis.

Research firms: Executive search firms and other agencies often employ research firms (sometimes their own) to identify potential candidates for positions. Sometimes it's the research firms that make initial contact with a candidate and the recruiter actually takes over at a later point in the process.

Corporate recruiters: Also called in-house recruiters, corporate recruiters are employed by one company and work on behalf of that company to find qualified candidates to fill the company's positions. Corporate recruiters are generally paid as salaried employees or hourly contractors, although they can sometimes receive bonuses for filling positions.

When you're speaking with a recruiter, it pays to know what type of recruiter they are—corporate, agency, research, executive search, etc. You should be comfortable asking them about their role and where they are in the search process. Before giving your resume to an agency, you should find out (and even get in writing) exactly where they intend to submit your resume. Once your resume has been submitted to a company through an agency you may be unable to submit your resume on your own for some period of time. If the client really wasn't an actual client but just a "potential" client, you may be left in a stalemate situation with an employer who wants to interview you and can't or won't pay the agency fee.

When contacted by a recruiter, you should also ask if he or she is calling about a specific opportunity, a future opportunity, or general career opportunities with a particular employer. If it's an executive search agency and they have a current search underway for which you're a fit, then it's a serious conversation. If they've seen your resume on a job board and think you might be a fit for upcoming positions at one or more client firms, then the conversation isn't quite as serious.

According to Patricia Nygren, MBA, a corporate recruiter in Roseville, California, and former Senior Employment Manager at Cisco Systems, Inc., some candidates think of recruiters as roadblocks. That isn't the case! "We want to fill the position and will always look for ways to rule a candidate 'in' rather than rule a candidate 'out,'" says Nygren. Recruiters are like sellers' agents in real estate—they work for the company, not for the candidate. Candidates sometimes forget this and think it's a recruiter's responsibility to find them a job or to give them career advice.

The hiring process is very time-intensive. With the advent of Internet job sites, email, and company Web sites, a recruiter can receive hundreds of resumes a day. They will pay more attention to resumes that are well written and easy to read. Candidates should do their best to make their resumes attractive to an employer. Explain gaps in job history if you've made lots of job changes. Also state if you're willing to relocate, if you've just relocated, etc. You can use a cover letter or summary section to highlight skills specific to a position. It's unlikely that a recruiter will take the time to go back and ask you for clarification.

Certain positions have very specific requirements or budget constraints. Even if you're the brightest new grad on the planet, a recruiter won't be able to hire you for a senior-level position, and vice versa. If the position is budgeted for a junior-level hire, they can't fill it with someone earning twice as much, even if you're willing to take a position with less responsibility.

According to Nygren, most recruiters always assume that candidates are on their best behavior during the interview process and that any behavioral red flags uncovered during the interviews will only be magnified once that person starts work. Recruiters are a key player in employers' decision-making process, so treat them with respect and be considerate of their time. Here are some typical questions about recruiters and the answers I received from both healthcare and high-tech recruiters.

How do you find a recruiter?

If a candidate makes a cold call, that starts the ball rolling. Depending on time and their communication skills, a recruiter may try to determine right then and there if there is a current opening that is an appropriate match. If there is a match, the recruiter will ask the caller to email a resume. After it is reviewed by the recruiter, a decision is made whether it fits any current positions. If so, it is forwarded to a manager, and the candidate is informed that a referral has occurred. If there is no match, the candidate is told that as well. If there might be future interest, the resume will likely be stored in a tickler file.

If you want to meet a recruiter, how do you find one?

Sutzi McGovern, MBA, a self-employed technical recruiter with more than 12 years' experience in recruiting with such firms as Cisco Systems, Inc., and Farmers Insurance Group, suggests asking friends or family. Nygren also suggests using your networking skills. Ask friends who placed them in particular jobs. Go to job fairs to meet corporate recruiters. Call a company and ask to speak with someone in recruiting. It doesn't hurt to send a resume even if there is not an exact match at the time, especially if it's a company you are targeting. Some Web sites have recruiters' email addresses. Generally, though, recruiters will come find you. Never pay for a recruiter. It is acceptable to pay to have your resume done professionally, but it's really not necessary unless you can't type and have no access to a computer or printer.

How do you know if a recruiter is reputable?

Ask for references. Check the Internet. Other candidates will be able to tell you, and trust your intuition. If a recruiter seems slimy, he or she probably is! Agency recruiting involves sales, just like cars, real estate, or insurance, except that both clients and products are people. There are reputable recruiters working for companies that may not be reputable. If you know someone in a job you want, ask that person how he or she got the job.

Do recruiters give career/resume/interview advice to you?

It depends on the recruiters' volume of work. McGovern says, "If I have the time, I do all of the above. If I have developed a rapport (usually by doing a phone interview) with them and think they may be a match, I will give them interview hints. If I see it's just naiveté on their part, I do give them resume advice even if I'm not bringing them in for an interview."

Nygren counters those comments with these thoughts:

As a corporate recruiter, I generally want to see how a candidate does on their own without coaching. An executive recruiter on a retained search has the luxury of a longer hiring cycle and also has more at stake, so might spend considerable time coaching an executive candidate on who they'll be meeting and what the hiring managers are looking for. An executive recruiter will also likely rewrite your resume to put in a presentation-style format. That being said, as a corporate recruiter, I'm happy to answer questions from candidates about who they'll be meeting, what to wear for the interview, etc. You should also ask questions of the recruiter and the hiring manager about the company and especially about what the key success factors for this particular position and/or employer are. The answers should give you some big clues as to what topics might be covered in an interview.

Should you ask a recruiter for his/her input on a specific job?

It is okay to ask any recruiter about the position. However, most of them aren't necessarily familiar with the specifics of the position or the technical aspects of a particular job—that's for the hiring manager and others on the team to discuss.

Should you contact a recruiter if you hear about a job you want?

Different companies have different rules about letting candidates through. It is always a good idea to try, especially with corporate recruiters. If you are dealing with agency recruiters, contact them only if you are certain that a particular agency or search firm is doing the hiring for the position you want.

Is recruiting at the executive/senior management level any different than at the mid-management/director level?

Definitely. At the executive level, there is almost always an executive search firm involved. And, as a rule, the hiring process takes longer the higher up you go in an organization. The candidates are usually known entities being convinced to join a company. There is more wooing then because the candidates have a known track record. If you're working with an executive search firm, you might have multiple interviews with the recruiter and/or research firm before even being presented as a candidate to the client.

Should a recruiter make comments about whether you should take a job or not?

The recruiters I interviewed don't believe that's the role of a recruiter. However, some recruiters discuss with candidates whether this is the right job for them. It may be more the company culture that may not match or a certain manager. Some recruiters believe recruitment is a two-way street and that the company and job should be right for the candidate. Whether you are working with a corporate or agency recruiter, the client is usually the employer, not the candidate. Candidates should know what's important to them in a job and do their best to ask appropriate questions during the interview in order to determine the fit with a particular employer and/or position.

Is it appropriate to work around a recruiter and talk directly to facility staff?

Usually what happens is the staff member will forward the resume or phone call to the recruiter. Very rarely will a candidate get an interview this way. If the candidate is a friend or family member of an executive or someone in senior management, the candidate may be given a courtesy interview, but this is very rare. Unless you've been told otherwise by a recruiter or by someone on the staff, I think it's okay to use your personal contacts within an organization to try to find a job. But once you've been told that you need to deal with the recruiter, you need to do so.

What if a recruiter tells you a job is one thing and it is actually something else?

Let the recruiter know that his or her information was incorrect about the position. Sometimes it's not the recruiter's fault that the information is bad—sometimes the employer hasn't given out the best information or there might have been a miscommunication during the interview process. The interview should give you the best idea of the job. It's always good practice to interview even if the job isn't right for you. Also, sometimes the criteria change from when the interview was set up until the interview is actually conducted.

What if you are recruited and hired, but the job is a bad fit?

Talk to your manager or the recruiter. Depending on how long it's taken the candidate to realize the bad fit, there may be something that can be done. If it's because of performance issues, the hired candidate may be fired. A corporate recruiter starts over and fills the position again. Agency contracts usually have a replacement clause where a portion of the fee is refunded or a replacement candidate is provided.

How is the recruiter affected by a bad hire?

Unless every candidate turns out not to be a good fit, not much happens. In most companies, the final decision to hire is with the managers and their teams. If they are

making a lot of bad hires, the recruiter usually steps in and does some interview training or assesses what the real issues are with the Human Resources partner.

How are recruiters paid?

Corporate recruiters are paid a salary no matter how many hires they create. If they
don't meet goals, that shortfall is reflected in their performance reviews. If they are on
contract, it may not be renewed. Agency recruiters are either on contingency or
retained. If they are on contingency, they get a specified percentage of the annual gross
salary after the candidate has been employed, usually after 90 days. Retained recruiters
are usually hired for executive searches and have contracts that pay them a certain
amount during all the different stages of the search.

Should you talk to recruiters even if you aren't looking for a job?

If contacted by a recruiter, you should always be gracious because you never know
when you'll need their services. Get their name and number and keep them on file for
the future. If they pester you, tell them not to call—they're probably not someone you
want to work with anyway. If you're not interested in a particular position but know
someone who is, give them that person's name or take their name to give to your friend.
Recruiting is all about networking, and what you put out there can come back to help
you in a very big way. If you talk to them when you don't want to, they are more likely
to remember and will talk to you when you need a job. That day always comes. Also
you may be able to refer a friend who's looking for a job, and that's a win-win.

For Your Toolkit

Create a relationship with at least one recruiter. You never know
when you will need one!

Chapter 4
General Career Skills

Important Job Skills

When interviewing for any position, keep in mind that in addition to technical and professional skills, employers are also looking for other skills. These other skills are often called "soft skills" (Vogt, 2005). Remember the phrase from your childhood report card, "works and plays well with others"? They were talking about a critical soft skill, and there are many more, all of them important for any job in any industry, but particularly in health care. There are numerous books and articles about these skills, with different names and labels. Essentially, these are the ones most cited (Vogt, 2005):

- Oral/spoken communication skills.
- Written communication skills.
- Being truthful and having integrity.
- Working effectively with others to accomplish tasks.
- Self-motivation/initiative—doing things without needing to be told or persuaded.
- Work ethic/dependability—being thorough and accurate so others can count on you.
- Critical thinking—challenging things when appropriate and proposing alternatives.
- Risk-taking skills—taking a considered chance on something new, different, or unknown.
- Flexibility/adaptability—going with the flow and adjusting to unforeseen circumstances.
- Influencing skills—persuading others to think about or adopt a different point of view.

- Organization skills—being organized and methodical, especially in work-related situations.
- Problem-solving skills—analyzing the potential causes of a problem and creating a solution.
- Multicultural skills—understanding and relating to people who are different from you.
- Computer skills—using basic word-processing, spreadsheet, and presentation software as well as the Internet.
- Academic/learning skills—learning new things quickly, thoroughly, and being willing to learn continuously.
- Making sure that even the little things are done and done correctly.
- Teaching/training skills—showing other people how to do something in a way that allows them to learn quickly and clearly.
- Guiding and supporting others in order to accomplish something.
- Relating to other people and communicating with them in everyday interactions.
- Handling the stress that accompanies deadlines and other limitations or constraints.
- Asking questions in order to learn or clarify something.
- Having the imagination to come up with new or out-of-the-box ideas.
- Quantitative skills—compiling and using numbers to study an issue or answer a question.
- Research skills—gathering information to answer questions.
- Time management skills—using your time wisely and consistently staying on schedule and meeting deadlines.

For Your Toolkit

> **Soft job skills are just as important as clinical competencies.**

Selling Yourself with No Experience

One of the biggest challenges in the workplace is selling yourself without having experience. How do people new to the job market land that first job with little or no real-world work experience? What can you do to jump-start your career if all you have is a brand-new diploma and a couple of unrelated summer jobs? Paul Barada (2005) believes that what you have to sell is job performance potential, and that's what you need to highlight. Here are some useful tips he offers on how to do just that.

A positive, upbeat, eager, self-confident attitude is critical. However, self-confidence should never be confused with arrogance or smugness. A can-do attitude is fine; that's what you want to radiate during the entire interview process. Demonstrate your willingness to take an entry-level position. Even with a degree, a lack of job experience normally means an entry-level position is all you can expect. In fact, an entry-level position is the ideal place to demonstrate your ability to learn quickly, pay your dues, and exceed your employer's expectations. Entry-level positions are a great opportunity for you to learn the job. Until you do, you aren't really valuable to an employer. The quicker you can learn the business of nursing and health care, the quicker you can expect to move up within the organization.

Demonstrate your desire to learn. Many people fail to make the clear distinction between classroom theory and real-world practice. Realize there is still much you don't know, not just about the job but also the organizational culture and politics, and the day-to-day reality of how things work.

Have reasonable salary expectations. Many new job seekers think there's a correlation between industry average salaries and their personal salary expectations. Some nurses are on a hunt for the job that pays the most money. Because signing bonuses are common in this field, candidates are often weeded out who appear to want to join the company simply for the signing bonus and leave shortly thereafter. Every company is different, and each has different compensation philosophies and policies. Also every new employee brings a different set of skills, training, experience, and ability to the job.

Be sure to focus on and highlight your soft skills. When employers are asked to rank the three most important skills they look for in new hires, they consistently identify the following: problem-solving skills, interpersonal skills, and the ability to work effectively with others in a team setting. Make a point to highlight those particular soft skills, including others you have, such as leadership, team-building, or communication—all of which are transferable from one job to another.

Don't rely on just your degree. Academic credentials are terrific, but they are not all that is needed in the employment setting. A degree is often used to screen job candidates in or out of the prospect pool. The degree signifies the completion of the coursework required. It is usually not an automatic pass into a spectacular first job. Some job seekers see their degree as an entitlement, not as a way to generate opportunities. A degree won't get you a job—it just opens the door.

For Your Toolkit

 A degree won't get you a job—it just opens the door.

With limited work experience, all you really can expect is the chance to prove what you can do. Your job-performance potential is the product you have to sell. In return, you can expect the chance to fulfill that potential. To expect more is to invite frustration and failure. Once your career is underway, your past job performance will speak for itself.

What Your Boss Wants You to Know

There are certain basic social and political skills required in virtually every job. These are the things your boss wishes you knew even if s/he hasn't told you. The survival skills are specific to work settings. If you know them, it is likely to be one reason you have been successful in your present job. In most workplaces, these skills are not spelled out explicitly. Even if you think they are obvious, consider all the people who don't know that—especially some of your fellow employees.

Come to Work

Regularly using all your sick time marks you as an outsider. Everyone is sick once in a while, but regularly missing a day or two here and there, especially on Mondays and Fridays, will label you as someone who doesn't have a clue about what it takes to be perceived as productive in your facility.

Identify with Your Facility

Speak and behave as if what's good for the facility is good for you. Think twice before you complain to other staff members or your boss. If you act as if your boss is your adversary, you are asking for trouble. You are also displaying the perception that your own problems with authority are more important to you than your job.

Watch Your Boss

Observe how your boss dresses, behaves in meetings, uses her/his time, or talks to employees (including you). Learn your boss's priorities and follow them. It doesn't matter if they seem wrong to you. Succeeding at your job often depends on seeing it from your boss's point of view rather than your own. If you have a boss who displays behaviors that you see are perceived as unacceptable by fellow employees or higher-level administrators, take note of that as well. You can always learn what *not* to do at the same time you are learning what to do.

Maintain a Professional Appearance

Every facility has its own standards for dress and a dress code. It is best to conform to it. A rule of thumb for dressing at work if you do not need to meet specific standards is not to wear anything that will call attention to you. Following the dress code does not mean you can't have your own style. Using your style within the confines of the dress standards will identify you as both conforming and creative.

Be Pleasant

Make an effort to get along with folks you work with. If you are upset with someone, try to deal calmly, courteously, and directly with that person. Don't take your problems to everyone you interact with. Eliminate eyeball-rolling and big frowns. Do your best to avoid participating in squabbles with co-workers—it will ruin your professional image.

Accept Direction and Criticism

It's great if your boss is specific and positive with her/his feedback. But work is like poker. You need to play the hand you're dealt.

Do Your Job as If It Were Worth Doing

Make it a point to learn all you can about your job and what it involves. Give your best effort to all parts of your job. It's a bad idea to make your boss remind you about the things you are not doing well.

Have a Sense of Humor

No one likes to work with people who take themselves too seriously. Keep a sense of humor about politics, illnesses, pets, and children.

For Your Toolkit

Survival advice:

- **Come to work.**
- **Identify with your facility.**
- **Watch your boss to identify priorities.**
- **Look professional.**
- **Be pleasant.**
- **Take direction and criticism gracefully.**
- **Do your job well.**
- **Have a sense of humor.**
- **Let go of vibrating poles.**

Turner Healthcare Associates, Inc., © 1994.

Let Go of Vibrating Poles

There are multiple issues in healthcare organizations that can make you crazy. Our natural tendency as nurses is to try and control things so we can "fix" them. Many healthcare facilities are dysfunctional, and we can't change much, if anything. As we continue to try and control whatever is dysfunctional, the more frustrated we get, and still not much changes. A healthcare organization is the equivalent of a vibrating pole. The temptation is to hang on to the pole to make it stop vibrating. In reality, that makes both you and the pole vibrate. The answer is to let go of the pole. Not easy to do in work settings, but it can be the only thing that will save your sanity.

Time Management

> *"The past is gone—the future may never be and all we have of the present is an invisible instant that is gone before we can say it is here."*

Even if you are not a manager, you can use ideas and tools to better manage time. More effective management of your time can mean that you have more time in your personal life to do the things you enjoy. These organizing skills will give you better time management as well as methods to better organize your energy and resources.

Time management is not about the amount of time we have. It is how we use the time that is available to us. Most people believe they do not have control of their time. When consistently applied, time-management skills will assist you in maximizing your time to achieve your personal and professional goals. Time is without a doubt our most valuable resource. Yet in spite of its preciousness, there is hardly anything else that we squander so thoughtlessly.

For Your Toolkit

Time management is not about the amount of time we have. It is how we use the time that is available to us.

Time has special characteristics. You can't accelerate its speed nor can you slow it down. You can't store it or recover time you have lost. Time is a gift that you cannot buy or sell. It cannot be controlled. Time simply slips away endlessly and relentlessly 1,440 minutes every day no matter who you are or what you do. Because of these characteristics, one of the measures of your success is how well you manage or invest your time. Time management is an individual activity, and the nurses who manage their time well are usually the best.

There are many reasons why people don't manage their work time well. Consider the ones that apply to you:

- There are too many uncontrollable interruptions.
- I am a pressure worker who produces best when faced with short schedules.
- I delay things I don't like to do.
- I don't plan; I react.
- I am usually too tired and have too little time to think about how I should spend my time.
- I am too preoccupied.
- I don't like my job.
- I have health problems.
- I am a perfectionist and never plan enough time for a project.
- I have too many chance meetings in the halls.
- I don't know how to manage my time.
- Others don't manage their time well and impose on me.
- I have too many demands.
- Managing my time is boring and too mechanistic.
- I can't prioritize because everything seems important.
- Time management is not possible.
- I don't delegate well.
- I am a procrastinator.
- I manage by crisis.
- I don't have adequate support.
- I have to attend too many meetings.
- There is too little communication.
- I am often confused about what tasks I should do.
- I don't have any goals.

These barriers and excuses keep you from managing your time effectively. You have more time when you practice time management. You can't change the way you have managed your time in the past, but you can manage your present opportunities better and plan for the future.

Nurses as well as nurse managers must focus on their daily priorities to enable them to reach their overall objectives. They must constantly organize themselves and their time.

Effective time management skills for nurses and nurse managers include:

- Develop objectives and priorities.
- Analyze how you use your time.
- Have a results-oriented (outcomes-based) plan.
- Organize for achievement.
- Control unproductive deviations or time wasters.
- Follow-up with periodic reviews to see how effectively you have used your time.

Peter Drucker, a well-known management consultant and writer, believed that the key to effectiveness is to know where our time should be spent for the results we want (Marks, 1994). The Pareto Principle says that 80% of our results come from 20% of what we do. Therefore, it appears that we tend to spend 80% of our time on low-value activities. This means that we are not using our time for maximum outcomes or results.

When evaluating your current time-management approach, you need to consider these questions about what you do:

- Does it relate to my job objectives?
- What is the immediacy of what I am doing?
- Why am I doing it? Could others do it?
- Is the time I spend proportionately matched to the priorities of my responsibilities?

Make a list of the ten most common things you do in your job. Of those 10 listed activities, check the two items that yield 80% of your results and objectives. What priorities do these activities have in your day? Do you focus on them, or do you just fit them in when you can? It is important to review how your actual work flow may be getting in the way of your accomplishing your objectives. We all have the same amount of time; the difference is how we use it. Time is a constant factor. It's what you do with the time that matters. The key to excellence is self-management, not time management.

There are some people who get everything done. It is easy to assume that you will be needed more if you don't get everything done. This is a myth. Another myth is to think that you can do more than one thing at a time. Although multitasking is commonplace, it is tough to do more than one thing at a time and do them effectively. The biggest misconception about time management is that waiting for a crisis is a good way to prioritize. Although waiting for a crisis certainly creates lots of motivation (and possibly fear), good planning eliminates the need for putting out many fires. Being proactive causes you less work in the end because you avert the problems and time-consuming cleanup jobs.

Other challenges are for those individuals who are procrastinators or perfectionists. Many people are both. Those juggling dozens of daily tasks and desires will not get things done if they use the mantra "if something's worth doing, it's worth doing well." Actually, those who apply extreme perfectionism to almost everything they do are almost always underachievers. That is because they tend to take too much time on unimportant tasks and lose momentum for the really important things.

Successful nurses know how to apply a flexible standard to each task, depending on its value. When appropriate, they are not above doing a "quick and dirty" job. An example of this strategy would be scanning a professional journal instead of reading it word for word. The "quick and dirty" strategy usually relates to nonclinical tasks. *Don't use this method when carrying out clinical patient procedures.*

There are many things that are time wasters. They limit your effectiveness. You can form new habits for each time waster. Evaluate these time wasters and see which ones get in your way of managing your goals and priorities:

- Attending meetings that don't matter.
- Procrastinating often.
- Having too many phone conversations.
- Having drop-in visitors who interrupt you.
- Not having a specific plan for the day.
- Not having specific and measurable business goals.
- Spending most of your time on routine tasks and trivia.
- Having a desk/work area that is cluttered.
- Being indecisive.
- Routinely having afternoon drowsiness.
- Having to repeat instructions/directions to subordinates.
- Paperwork taking up a huge part of your day.
- Trying to do it all to be successful.
- Unexpected problems causing you to react and divert other priorities.
- Routinely joining the "coffee break" folks.
- Lacking specific time blocks to work on priorities.

Any of the above items that you recognize as your own behavior are limiting your effectiveness. Pick one area and minimize its effect as a time waster.

There are ways to gain time. You can incorporate them into your daily life to enable you to accomplish your personal and professional goals. Each one you implement will help you gain time:

- *Meetings:* Only hold meetings using an agenda. Start on time, be on time, and end on time. Delegate to others any meetings you can. Schedule meetings back to back.

- *Procrastination:* Set deadlines and specific priorities. Promise results in writing to another person. Break large projects into small ones.
- *Phone interruptions:* When working on top projects/issues, have calls screened or let voicemail pick up. Get out of your office. Limit time spent on routine phone calls.
- *Drop-in visitors:* Stand to talk to the visitor. Explain that you would love to talk but cannot do so now. Be direct but polite. Close your door when you are working.
- *Daily plan:* Use one that is simple. Every day, write down six things to do, in order of priority. Start with item 1 and work one at a time. Don't worry if you don't finish all the items. Transfer the unfinished items to the next day's list.
- *Goals:* Set business and personal goals. It works to help make you more productive. Lack of direction wastes time and effort. Goal-setting is one of the greatest success secrets of all time.
- *Routine and trivia:* Do routine or trivial things by a schedule. Don't do it just whenever it pops up. Save junk mail, phone calls, or reading for times you have less energy or for nonprime time.
- *Cluttered desk:* Clean off your desk, put anything you can out of sight so you are not distracted. Consider having only papers on your desk that represent priorities, for example, three or four.
- *Indecision:* Gather information and act. Take calculated risks, which is a manager's job. Keep others appropriately involved or informed of your decisions.
- *Giving directions:* Be specific, and if you need to, ask subordinates to paraphrase or repeat your instructions back to you. Always follow up to check results, and consider putting detailed or complex instructions in writing.
- *Paperwork:* Don't write memos; call whenever possible. Handle mail only once. Write notes on letters/memos and return them instead of doing another separate letter or memo. Any time you pick up a piece of paper, do something with it, including filing or throwing it away. Don't stack it up to "do something with later." I stand at the recycle bin to sort mail. Anything that is junk mail goes directly into the recycler and never comes into my office.
- *Afternoon drowsiness:* Take a walk at noon or work out in a health club. Eat a light lunch. Consider a short walk or a high-protein snack in the afternoon to counteract the drowsiness. Don't eat high-carbohydrate or high-sugar foods at lunch or for a snack.
- *Trying to do it all:* Focus on the 20% of your tasks that yield 80% of your results. Delegate to others whenever possible. Say "no" sometimes. Take a break occasionally. You will be more effective.
- *Unexpected problems:* Handle them swiftly if they are urgent. Don't fret or worry about what you have done. You can't be a prophet and plan for everything. Make sure you train and empower your staff to solve their own problems when they can.

Ask "what are *you* going to do?" Don't fix the problem yourself if the staff members can solve it on their own.

- *Coffee klatsches:* If you are committed to excellence and getting your job done, skip the coffee breaks. Be sociable after hours.
- *Interruptions:* When working on priorities, have your phone calls screened. Close your door or work in a different location. Establish quiet times and get things done during the day. You don't have to work longer hours to be effective.

There are several ways to gain time. Real time management is self-management. You can't manage time, but you can manage yourself. Time is constant, 168 hours per week. What you do with those hours is the secret to getting more done. One of the most efficient physicians I know says, "We all have the same twenty-four hours; I just choose to do more with mine."

To manage yourself better, you must be willing to change. New habits must replace old habits. Change is usually uncomfortable at first. With persistence and repetition, this can be overcome. The key to self-management is to manage your response to an event. Good time managers are good at controlling their responses to events they can't control. Use time-gaining techniques. How you respond to time wasters depends on your attitude and your willingness to plan.

You can create your own time analysis and develop a personal self-management program. Outline the objectives you want to accomplish each week. Prioritize those objectives according to their importance to you. Make sure you take some time out at the beginning or end of the day (for the next day) to do your daily to-do list. Review yesterday's list and create the next day's list. Make sure to highlight the tasks you must complete today. The time of day you plan depends on when you are most alert and have some quiet time to concentrate and reflect.

Be prepared for your to-do list strategy to be sabotaged and for things to get in the way. You should always plan on "Murphy's law" being in effect. This law is "whatever can go wrong, will go wrong." The other given is that everything always takes longer than you think. Keep in mind that there are three keys to managing time:

1. Assess time by determining if objectives are realistic in the time you allotted.
2. Set priorities so that what is important is what is accomplished.
3. Stick to your plan and be single-minded. Eliminate time-wasting habits.

If you are an effective supervisor, you know the abilities, initiatives, and dependability of each subordinate. Delegate accordingly. Reduce the routine order of things and schedule similar tasks together whenever possible.

Additional ideas for helping you become better organized include:

- Declutter your desk each day so that you are not losing documents and getting distracted.
- Consolidate similar tasks.
- Before making a call or visit, outline the basic points to be covered. On the telephone, identify yourself immediately and spend minimal time on chit chat. If a personal visit is necessary, make an appointment first.
- Delegate what is appropriate. Develop your subordinates' ability to assume routine tasks, plan, think creatively, and handle more responsibility to free you up for supervisory tasks.
- Plan concentrated time blocks for those projects and problems that need analysis and uninterrupted time. When you are interrupted, you often have to go back over material you covered before the interruption. Schedule a time to make and return phone calls.
- Avoid procrastination and work on priority items until you complete them.
- Practice clear and direct communication. Unclear directions and communication waste your and others' time by causing things to be redone and reexplained.
- Practice streamlined reading by finding central thoughts, major themes, and skimming materials. Read whole thoughts and phrases at a time to improve speed and comprehension.
- Sort your papers on your desk by using:
    i. *Toss*. If the paper has no value, don't keep it. Throw it away now; don't keep it to throw away later.
    ii. *Refer*. Pass papers onto subordinates or appropriate co-workers when possible. Write a note on the document to the person receiving it. Put it in the out box.
    iii. *Act*. A paper requiring a response from you should be put in an action file.
    iv. *File*. A paper that might have future value for you should be placed in a desk/cabinet file. If your file cabinets are a distance from your desk, stack all items to be filed together, and take them to the cabinet all at one time.
    v. Schedule a time each day to process/sort mail and answer it.
    vi. Keep track of complex, deferred, and referred actions with a calendar or index cards in a "holding status" file.
    vii. Make a quick desk check at the end of each day to be sure all papers have been sorted as above.
- Plan meetings carefully. They are good for generating ideas, sharing information, and making decisions that require group input.
- Call a meeting if you need to:
    i. define goals.

   ii. reach group judgments on decisions.
  iii. discover, analyze, or solve a problem.
   iv. gain acceptance for an idea, program, decision, or change.
    v. reconcile conflicting views.
   vi. provide essential information.
  vii. assure understanding of policy, methods, or decisions.
 viii. obtain immediate reactions when speedy responses to a problem are required.
- *Do not* use a meeting format if you:
    i. can communicate in another medium such as telephone, memo, or email and get results.
   ii. have insufficient time for adequate preparation.
  iii. discover that one or more key participants are not available.
   iv. find that the time is not convenient.
    v. think the net return on the cost of the meeting isn't realized.
- Make sure when you call a meeting that you:
    i. prepare for the meeting.
   ii. start and end on time!
  iii. get to the point.
   iv. watch group dynamics. Are people frustrated? Angry? Contributing? Complaining about wasting time?
    v. summarize accomplishments.
   vi. follow up with minutes and action items.
  vii. keep tabs on action-item progress.

Keep in mind as you try all these new techniques that it takes a minimum of 21 days to establish positive changes in behavior. Remember that the rewards for effective time management will come in both your professional and personal life and last a lifetime. Successful staff and managers have control of their time because they are organized for achievement.

Evaluate Your Communication Style: It Does Affect Your Career

There are numerous definitions for communication. It is an active process, not a static one. According to Bernard and Walsh (1996), communication is the sending and receiving of information, feelings, and attitudes, both verbally and nonverbally, to produce a response. In effective communication, a message is transmitted and received, but the real process of communicating starts when the receiver provides a response to the sender.

Effective communication occurs between two persons when the receiver interprets the sender's message the same way that the sender intended it. Both the sender and the receiver are affected by personal background, attitudes, perceptions, emotions, opinions, education, and experience. There is a specific meaning in the message the sender intends to send. There are also symbols used to communicate—both verbally and nonverbally. The message has no meaning until it is received.

A successful communication sequence looks like this:

Sender → Meaning → Message → Symbols → Meaning → Receiver

Essentially, this means that the same factors that create effective communication can also be barriers to effective communication. For example, a speaker's ethnic background can make that person great at communicating with other members of the same ethnicity; however, the speaker may not be equally as effective when speaking to an ethnically diverse audience (Turner, 1999).

Being insensitive can damage communication by causing the sender or receiver to look at the situation from only one point of view. Nonverbal gestures, movements such as tapping, avoiding eye contact, voice tone, pitch, inflection, and mumbling also cause ineffective communication.

Nurses can use strategies to improve communication and become successful at communication in the workplace. During stressful times, effective communication becomes critical. Because many nurses are often overwhelmed and frustrated, these strategies become even more important. Try using an open-ended style of questioning. Open-ended questions are questions requiring more than a "yes" or "no" answer. Select the proper environment to have your conversation. Offering criticism to a co-worker at the nurses' station is not only rude, but unkind. Privacy is an important consideration for nurses and patients, as well as anyone involved in conflict or a stress-producing situation.

Timing of communication is crucial. It may not be a good idea to bring up a conflict to your boss on a bad day or on his/her birthday. Be selective when choosing to discuss conflicts. Send your own message by using first-person singular pronouns and explanations ("I feel . . ."). This type of personal ownership includes clearly taking responsibility for the ideas and feelings that one expresses. People disown their messages when they use phrases like "most people" or "our group." This type of language

For Your Toolkit

Your timing of communication is crucial.

makes it difficult for listeners to tell whether the individuals really think and feel what they are saying or whether they are repeating the thoughts and feelings of others.

Ask for feedback on how your messages are received. To communicate effectively, you must be aware of how the receiver is interpreting and processing your messages. The only way to be sure is to seek feedback on what meanings the receiver is attaching to your messages. Make the message appropriate to the receiver's frame of reference. Use different appropriate words and depths of explanation for an expert in the field, a novice, a child, an adult, your boss, or a co-worker.

Nonverbal communication is the most important aspect of communication and often the most ignored. Body language is 55% of communication. Tone of voice is 38%. The actual words stated comprise only 7% of the communicated message (Bernard and Walsh, 1996). Maintaining good eye contact instills credibility and honesty in the receiver. Make verbal and nonverbal messages consistent and congruent. Every face-to-face communication involves both verbal and nonverbal messages. Usually these messages are congruent. Problems arise when a person's verbal and nonverbal messages are contradictory because the nonverbal messages do not support the verbal messages and the receiver is confused.

Make your messages complete and specific. Include clear statements of necessary information the receiver

The elements of communication are:

- the sender.
- the receiver.
- the message sent (the meaning the sender wants to send).
- symbols (how the message is sent, e.g., verbal, nonverbal).
- the message received (the meaning actually received).

Barriers to effective communication include:

- preconceived assumptions and stereotypes.
- distractions like extraneous noise, too many people talking at once.
- emotional triggers like judgmental statements or expression of feelings that create listener resentment and defensiveness, such as "What did you do now?"
- confusing or complex language that has a different meaning to sender and receiver, for example, "Did the patient void?"
- physical barriers, for example, hearing impairment.
- being unprepared.
- failure to be direct and concise.
- feelings of intimidation in a high-pressure environment.
- poor timing because the receiver is unable or not ready to listen (Turner, 1998).

needs in order to comprehend the message. Being complete and specific seems obvious, but often people do not communicate the frame of reference they are using, the assumptions they are making, the intentions they have in communicating, or the leaps in thinking they are making.

Focus on issues and behaviors, not people. Describe others' behavior without evaluating or interpreting. When reacting to the behavior of others, be sure to describe their behavior, for example, "You keep interrupting me," rather than evaluating it, for example, "You're a rotten, self-centered egotist who won't listen to anyone else's ideas." Get rid of excess baggage by concentrating on the basic communication experience. Learn to minimize redundancy, excessive detail, irrelevant information, and distractions. Outline in your mind what you want to say.

Listening is a critical element of the communication process. Listening skills can be developed. Anyone who wants to get the most from a dialogue must be both a good speaker and a good listener. Types of listening are defined as passive and active. Passive listening is listening that you don't have to work at, such as to TV and music. Active listening requires full attention in order to hear and understand the entire message.

For Your Toolkit

> Listening is critical to your success.

To be successful at active listening, you must listen for the purpose of understanding what is meant, not for the purpose of readying yourself for a reply. Try to listen to the whole message first: don't interpret too quickly what the speaker is trying to say. Attempt to put aside your own views and opinions while actively listening. Put yourself in the speaker's shoes, and try to understand how s/he views the world.

Try to keep your thoughts from being interrupted by how you plan to respond. Don't trust your intuition. Validate the message with the sender. Expect the speaker to use different words than you might use, and try not to make snap judgments about what you are hearing. There are different styles of communication that work in different situations. It is important for nurses to be familiar with and competent in all these types of communication.

Chapter 5
Nursing Roles

"Be the change that you want to see in the world."
—MAHATMA GANDHI

Nonclinical Nursing Roles in a Hospital

When providing bedside care loses its appeal, you can renew your energy for nursing by working in a nonclinical specialty. You can draw on your clinical experience and still love nursing. There are numerous jobs available for experienced nurses who are no longer able or willing to deliver bedside clinical nursing care. These jobs are few and far between, but most healthcare facilities have them. There are also nursing roles outside hospital settings available to experienced nurses.

Patient/Staff Educator

Clinical nurse educators help patients and their families understand the patient's condition prior to discharge, and what to do for the patient once they are all at home. Educators offer independent classes and they can also work in outpatient areas like cardiac rehabilitation, diabetes education, or childbirth preparation. In most facilities, clinical educators also orient and train new nurses and provide additional courses and inservice training for staff nurses. Clinical nurse educators possess at least a BSN. Some have advanced clinical training in a specialty.

They must be able to communicate clearly, and nurse educators must enjoy teaching. A passionate educator will get students or patients excited about the subject. Nurse educators need to be able to write education plans, organize courses, and have excellent time management and written and oral communication skills.

Quality Improvement

Nurses involved in quality improvement constantly ask the question, "How can this be improved or done better?" Nurses in this role review a healthcare institution's methods and processes. Their work is evidence-based and outcome-focused. By studying patient populations, they analyze systems to determine how to correct problems and improve quality of care. In short, they strive to prevent future problems by studying past mistakes (Mehallow, 2005).

Nurses in this role usually have a bachelor's degree in nursing or a related healthcare field. Being a certified professional in healthcare quality (CPHQ) is a definite plus, but not all employers require that certification. The Healthcare Quality Certification Board oversees CPHQ testing. In most facilities, nurses involved in quality improvement work in a department outside nursing that reports to a senior executive. Excellent written and oral communication skills are a must, along with political savvy and patience.

Risk Manager

Risk management is closely tied to quality improvement. Risk managers also search for the root causes of mistakes to help improve systems and processes. Nurses are great in this role because they already think about patients using the nursing process. Job opportunities for risk managers are increasing at hospitals and in all types of clinical settings. Even insurance companies and law practices use nurses in these roles. Risk-management nurses review patient records before and after lawsuits are filed and during legal proceedings. Risk managers work with senior medical and administrative staff. These jobs require patience, tact, and political savvy plus excellent communication, conflict resolution, and writing skills.

Most risk-management nurses hold at least a bachelor's degree and risk-management certification, which is available from the American Hospital Association Certification Center, the American Board of Quality Assurance and Utilization Review Physicians, and some colleges.

Case Manager

Case managers are the choreographers of the patient-care experience. They coordinate all the healthcare team members, ensuring continuity and that everyone understands what is happening with patients. As hospitals discharge patients more quickly, and managed-care organizations oversee patient care more closely, the need for case managers has increased. The aging population is generating more opportunities in long-term care and home health care as well (Mehallow, 2005).

More facilities are looking for nurses who have both strong clinical experience and certification in case management. The two primary certifying bodies are the Commission for Case Manager Certification and the American Nurses Credentialing Center. Case managers are expected to create the highest achievable patient outcome with the shortest possible hospitalization. This role requires nurses who are self-directed, proactive, and able to create change. Characteristics needed to be successful in this role include patience, diplomacy, and political astuteness.

Chart Auditor

Nurses often serve as financial chart auditors. The role requires review of patient charts after discharge to ensure appropriate documentation for proper billing and coding. Chart auditors also work in quality management and review charts for appropriate clinical documentation of all aspects of patient care, including nursing. Many chart auditors are ADN or diploma-holding nursing school grads. A graduate degree is not required by most facilities for this role. Chart auditors need excellent reading skills and the ability to communicate their findings to others. Political savvy is a plus, because folks in this role must ask other clinicians to improve or revise their chart documentation.

Patient Advocate

Nurses can also serve as patient advocates. This role is customer-service focused. Patient advocates primarily handle patient complaints. This is an excellent nursing role for a nurse with a physical disability that limits the active tasks of bedside nursing or a mature nurse who can no longer tolerate the physical demands of bedside nursing. No additional education or training is required for this role. Patient advocates need excellent listening skills, patience, and a solution-focused problem-solving perspective.

Preceptor

More and more hospitals are creating formal positions for experienced nurses to guide new nurses through the critical first year on the job. As hospitals recognize the connection between strong preceptor skills and new-grad retention rates, formal programs for training preceptors are being developed. Preceptors are experienced nurses who enjoy teaching and working with new nurses and new graduates. Patience is a must, plus a positive attitude, and the ability to make people feel comfortable asking questions. No additional nursing education is required for this role, although many hospitals require formal preceptor training before doing this type of work. This is a great role for an older nurse no longer able to perform bedside nursing care.

Clinical Information System Consultants

Many healthcare facilities are looking for nurses to assist in converting existing patient data systems to electronic medical record systems. Nurses' clinical knowledge and ability to understand all the steps in patient hospitalization make them perfect project coordinators. These roles require patience, technology knowledge, and the ability to work between the nursing and information-technology worlds. Political savvy is a plus, because in this role a nurse functions as a change agent and project champion. Additional education and training is usually not required.

Primary nursing education and clinical experience provide lots of options once a nurse determines that bedside nursing is no longer a viable career option. To assess these types of jobs, ask to job shadow with someone currently in the role to see if it is a fit for you.

Clinical Informatics Specialist

The hospital implementation of information technology has given nurses added responsibility throughout the country. However, it has also provided new professional specialties. Clinical informatics is one of them. These nurses are part of a clinical team that promotes patient care through the design, implementation, and maintenance of the hospital's clinical information system (DeRitis, 2004). Clinical systems usually interface with other hospital systems, like the pharmacy, ER, laboratory, and registration systems. These interfaces support clinical decision-making and are critical to patient-care issues. Nurses can fill these roles and assist with the development of these systems. Their clinical mentality becomes crucial in designing the finished product.

Technology is also advancing at the bedside, with many facilities implementing personal PDAs for nursing documentation, as well as bar-coding patient admission armbands and medications. These bedside advancements also involve clinical informatics specialists.

Nursing Roles in the Community

Mid-career nurses can reinvent themselves without starting over. Experienced nurses can apply their clinical skills and experience outside of the hospital. Take a look at these career possibilities. One of them may allow you to realign or rediscover your passion for nursing.

Correctional Nursing

There are 2 million inmates and juvenile offenders behind bars in this country. Nurses who work with them deal with a range of medical problems, from toothaches to trauma. Most inmates do not have easy access to health care. Correctional nurses enjoy taking care of people who need a lot of services and education. The biggest challenge of correctional nursing is the ability to look at people not by what they have done, but for who they are. This is not a role for everyone, but those who do it, love it.

Correctional nurses work autonomously. They assess new inmates, manage the chronic diseases and mental illnesses of long-term prisoners, and respond to acute illnesses and injuries. These nurses must be confident, mature, and well-rounded. Nursing in prisons and jails is safe, because guards are always nearby and the environments are carefully controlled. No additional educational credentials are required, but training on how to work in a correctional setting is provided on the job. Patience, excellent communication skills, and a nonjudgmental attitude are musts for this role.

Forensic Nursing

Nurses have always worked with victims and perpetrators of violent crime, but it wasn't until the early 1990s that forensic nursing became a common description for this work. Now, there are almost 8,000 registered nurses who regularly fill forensic-nursing roles. Forensic nurses assess crime victims and perpetrators to look for even the smallest sign of injury to show whether an assault did or did not occur. Some work full time investigating deaths or treating violent offenders at psychiatric facilities and others moonlight as Sexual Assault Nurse Examiners (SANE) or legal nurse consultants (Mehallow, 2005).

Hollywood's portrayal of forensic nursing in shows such as *CSI* is misleading. Forensic nurses must be patient, methodical, and thorough in their assessments in order to provide evidence that can withstand the scrutiny of a court.

Additional specialty training is required for this role. Nurses who are interested in this field can get a taste of forensic nursing by participating in one of 400 SANE training programs offered at hospitals and other sites around the country (Mehallow, 2005).

Holistic Nursing

Holistic nursing is a growing specialty. Healthcare consumers' acceptance of the philosophy that treating the whole person is better than treating just a disease or symptom has caused this field to expand exponentially in the last decade. Improved insurance coverage for alternative healthcare practices has also allowed more patients to explore this care option. Any nurse who practices holism embraces the mind/body/spirit connection and empowers patients to participate in their own healing.

In addition to embracing the holistic philosophy, many nurses become proficient and earn certification or licensure in such other healing modalities as therapeutic massage, aromatherapy, imagery, herbology, or Reiki. These practices complement Western medicine and are frequently encouraged by traditional physicians. Whereas some practitioners work full-time nursing jobs and practice their healing modality on the side, others take positions in holistic wellness centers, spas, health clubs, and physicians' offices. Additional education is required to practice in this specialty (Mehallow, 2005).

Parish Nursing

The most important role of a parish nurse is helping people understand how faith and health work together. Parish nurses promote healthful living by educating and counseling parishioners on exercise and nutrition, advocating for community health, helping sick parishioners navigate the medical system, and developing support groups for bereavement, parenting, divorce, and other issues.

Most parish nurse roles are unpaid. The paid ones usually work 20 hours or less per week. Nurses interested in this specialty should work with their own churches to get started or investigate whether any local hospitals sponsor parish-nurse outreach programs. There is usually no additional training required for this specialty. Many retired nurses seek these roles to continue nursing while serving the community (Mehallow, 2005).

Legal Nurse Consulting

Legal nurse consultants work at the crossover between medicine and law, consulting with attorneys and others in the legal arena on medical malpractice, personal injury, workers' compensation, and other healthcare-related cases. The legal nurse consultant's main function is educating attorneys, to whom these nurses are a huge asset. Many legal nurse consultants work on the staff of law firms, insurance companies, and other institutions. Others work independently, charging an hourly fee for their work. Legal nurse consulting allows nurses to branch out from the clinical setting while still making use of their experience and knowledge. The functions of a legal nurse consultant include interviewing clients, reviewing medical records, researching and summarizing medical literature, assisting with the evaluation of liabilities and damages, assisting with depositions, preparing exhibits, and working with expert witnesses.

Independent legal nurse consultants perform many of the same tasks as their in-house counterparts. In addition, they sometimes serve as expert witnesses at depositions or trials, where they are called upon to testify about nursing deviations from established standards of care. Many independent legal nurse consultants still work full or part time in the hospital. The demand is higher for independent legal nurse consultants currently working in the field who can offer the most informed opinions on nursing issues.

The field of legal nurse consulting has grown tremendously and there are now thousands of legal nurse consultants in practice across the nation. The only prerequisite to becoming a legal nurse consultant is clinical experience. Many legal nurse consultants have backgrounds in critical, intensive, and emergency care. Although formal training in legal nurse consulting is not required to practice, training and educational programs are available at universities, community colleges, nonprofits, and for-profit organizations.

Healthcare Consultant

Does it sound exciting to strike out on your own? Many nurses carve out lucrative niches as consultants, offering data analysis, strategic planning, project management, or architectural services. Besides health and methodology expertise, consultants must have the ability to communicate in a way that the client understands. Nurses need to understand and have a feel for the client's content area. You must be able to market and sell your services. That includes managing relationships, negotiating and closing a deal, estimating jobs accurately, and figuring out market-rate pricing.

Consultants need to identify a broad area in which to specialize. Failing to be specific about your area of expertise limits your credibility, but not being broad enough can pigeon-hole you into only consulting about certain things. You must also have an alternative source of income for six months to one year because it takes that long to generate clients and a consistent revenue stream from consulting. Keep in mind that there is usually a time lag between getting a referral and actually starting the work. You need to have a plan for income during the time lag.

Medical Office Manager

Nurses are well suited to run a physician's office, a hectic job requiring a wide range of skills and constant multitasking. HIPAA, OSHA, and compliance laws make this position much more complex than in the past. Office managers must understand billing and coding as well as clinical-care issues. This is a great role for a nurse no longer able to handle the physical aspects of bedside nursing.

The Professional Association of Health Care Office Management, the Practice Management Institute, and the Association of Registered Health Care Professionals offer certification programs for office managers. While most office managers learn on the job, some community colleges now offer associate's degrees in healthcare office management (Mehallow, 2005).

Research Nurse

Research nurses are the eyes, ears, and hands that conduct much of today's clinical research. Staff research nurses participate in clinical trials that evaluate new drugs and medical devices. They work with the principal investigator and research coordinators. They evaluate potential studies, screen and schedule patients, coordinate patient visits according to protocols, review patient progress, and help report study results.

Research nurses can also conduct research related to the practice of nursing. They may evaluate and study nursing care practices, procedures, or care philosophies with the sole purpose of improving nursing practice.

Research nurses typically work in academic medical centers, educational institutions, pharmaceutical companies, and private research foundations, but private-practice physicians are now also hiring research nurses. Most research positions require a master's degree (Mehallow, 2005).

Case Manager

Distinct from those managers who coordinate hospital patient care, case managers also work for managed-care companies, home-care agencies, nursing agencies, and management-services organizations to minimize duplication of care and services and maximize clinical and financial outcomes.

These nurses must understand Medicare/Medicaid regulations, managed-care guidelines, and the care guidelines issued by the Joint Commission on Accreditation of Healthcare Organizations. Case managers also must be proficient in criteria issued by InterQual and Millman & Robertson, two leading developers of level-of-care guidelines (Mehallow, 2005).

Telemedicine Nurse

These are nurses who interact with patients via phone or the Internet. They advise managed-care subscribers based on physician-developed protocols. Academic medical centers often employ nurses as research assistants to perform telephone consultations with patients participating in clinical trials. Additional academic preparation is usually not required (Mehallow, 2005).

Cruise-Ship Nurse

Cruise ships now have floating medical centers on board. These on-board care centers resemble urgent care centers and have state-of-the-art equipment, much like an ER. Nurses see patients in the center and in cabins if patients are too sick to make it to the medical center. They administer medications, monitor chronic illnesses, and treat emergencies. This role is great for nurses who like to travel and enjoy ER, ICU, and urgent-care nursing. ER experience is usually required, but additional academic preparation is not needed.

Pharmaceutical and Medical-Equipment and Supply Educators

These nurses educate hospital staff members and physicians on using new medical equipment, supplies, and pharmaceuticals. Clinical experience in hospitals is usually required, but no additional academic preparation is necessary. This kind of role usually requires extensive travel.

School Nursing

If you love working with children and want your summers off, consider school nursing. School nurses do screenings, educate in classrooms, treat sick children, and handle emergencies. School nurses also work with teachers, administrators, and parents. A BSN is required in most states as well as additional training. Most school nurses routinely multitask and are responsible for several schools at a time. This is a great role if you are self-directed and independent.

Occupational Nursing

Occupational- and environmental-health nursing is the specialty practice that provides for and delivers health and safety programs and services to workers, worker populations, and community groups. The practice focuses on promotion and restoration of health, prevention of illness and injury, and protection from work-related and environmental hazards.

In the past two centuries, their responsibilities have expanded immensely to encompass a wide range of job duties, including case management, counseling and crisis intervention, health promotion, legal and regulatory compliance, and worker and workplace hazard detection.

Typically, nurses entering the field have a BSN and experience in community health, ambulatory care, critical care, or emergency nursing. Certification in occupational- and environmental-health nursing is highly recommended.

Broadcast Journalist

Nurses can also choose a broadcasting career. Television healthcare reporter roles are often filled by nurses. Most nurses in these roles have many years of experience in nursing and are specialists in at least one area of health care. A master's degree is helpful but not mandatory. This role is a great way to bring your passion for nursing to the public.

Architectural Building Design/Construction Management

Nurses who enjoy working with building construction may have a career niche here. Participating in the design of new medical facilities allows nurses to use their clinical mentality, as well as learn skills in the field of architecture and construction management. Assisting architects and construction project managers, nurses can help identify patient flow, systems design, operations logistics, and other aspects of building development. These types of positions usually require several years of clinical nursing experience. Nurses can be used as consultants or hired by architectural firms. Nurses can also attend architect programs and become certified as architects, specializing in healthcare facilities.

Nursing Education

RNs with master's or doctoral degrees are in great demand as faculty at nursing schools. The current nursing faculty shortage, which the AACN reports at 8.1% nationally, is a major contributor to the shortage of all types of nurses. Nursing schools turned away more than 32,000 qualified applicants in 2004 due to a shortage of faculty and resources, according to the AACN (Rossheim, 2005). Being a nurse educator allows you to shape the nursing profession and share your skills and expertise with others.

Nurses with lots of clinical experience have very important skill perspectives that students and new graduates need to have. More faculty members will be required in the future. The shortage of nursing educators is expected to worsen in coming years as many faculty members retire. According to AACN survey data released in March 2005, 65% of the nearly 11,000 faculty members teaching in the nation's bachelor's and graduate nursing programs were over 50 (Rossheim, 2005).

Clinical experience is a key element of nursing education, which means nurses who teach don't have to give up patient contact. Teaching in a nursing baccalaureate program does mean earning an advanced degree. Many nurses can find ways to earn an advanced degree without entirely giving up their clinical practice income. Scholarships, forgivable loans, and tuition-reimbursement programs are all ways to finance becoming a nurse educator. Financial aid for nurses attending graduate school is available from many sources, including the federal and state governments, hospitals and other healthcare employers, nursing associations, and nursing schools.

There are online programs that enable nurses to fit graduate study into their lives while continuing to work. Perhaps the most difficult obstacle for nurses aspiring to be professors is the salary cut they're likely to experience at the start of their academic careers. The average salary of an ER nurse practitioner with a master's degree was nearly $81,000, versus about $60,000 for a nursing professor with the same academic training, according to a 2003 survey by *Advance for Nurse Practitioners* magazine (Rossheim, 2005). However, as they move up the academic ladder, faculty members with doctoral degrees earn well into six figures.

Advanced-Practice Nursing Roles

If you are an experienced nursing professional, there are a number of opportunities in advanced-practice nursing you can pursue. There are four categories of advanced-practice nurses: nurse practitioner (NP), certified registered nurse anesthetist (CRNA), certified nurse midwife (CNM), and clinical nurse specialist (CNS). All require advanced education (typically a master's degree) and clinical experience. After that, certification and state licensing requirements vary.

Nurse Practitioners

Nurse practitioners (NPs) must hold a master's degree and a state license. They are in short supply in many parts of the country and may be an area's only source of primary care, especially in rural settings. NPs often provide primary health care. Their responsibilities include:

- conducting physicals.
- making diagnoses and providing treatment.
- writing prescriptions.
- managing patients' chronic conditions, such as diabetes and hypertension.

NPs must be knowledgeable about prescription medications and be self-directed and self-reliant. They must also know when to call in a physician for consultation or to take over the care of a seriously ill patient. NPs can own their practices or work in hospitals, managed-care organizations, and clinics. To work with physicians in a private-practice setting or establish a practice of your own, consider specializing in areas such as women's health or gerontology.

Certified Registered Nurse Anesthetists

Certified registered nurse anesthetists (CRNAs) are among the most highly educated and highly compensated of advanced nurse professionals. In addition, some states are allowing CRNAs to practice without physician supervision. CRNAs work in all settings, from hospitals to private offices. Most states require CRNAs to hold an MSN from an accredited program in the field. CRNAs must also be licensed and certified in their state of practice.

Certified Nurse Midwives

Certified nurse midwives (CNMs) provide prenatal and gynecological care to women, deliver babies, and provide postpartum care. Most midwife-attended births still occur in hospitals, but CNMs also practice in birthing centers and oversee home births. Many work as solo practitioners or in partnership with an OB/GYN or other CNMs. Most states require CNMs to be RNs, as well as hold a master's degree.

Clinical Nurse Specialists

A clinical nurse specialist (CNS) is an expert in a specialized area of clinical nursing. A CNS can specialize in a specific disease (such as cancer), population (such as women or children), setting (such as an ER), type of care (such as rehab), or type of problem (such as pain) (Rossheim, 2005). A CNS requires a master's or doctorate and certification to practice as a CNS, and many are also nurse practitioners.

Chief Nursing Executives

Another option for registered nurses is to move into the executive suite. As the choreographer of patient care, no one knows better about how all the ancillary services support patient-care needs. Nurses in the chief nurse executive (CNE) role usually serve as nurse managers and directors before taking this type of role. A master's degree in fields such as nursing, healthcare administration, or business is required. Some chief nurse executives move on to become chief executive or chief operating officers, overseeing the entire healthcare organization. Who better to run the place than an RN?

Chapter 6
Supervision and Management Skills

Portrait of a Leader

- Persistence. Not insistence. A strong leader hangs on a little longer, works a little harder.
- Imagination. S/he harnesses imagination to practical plans that produce results.
- Vision. The present is just the beginning. A good leader is impressed with the possibilities of the future.
- Sincerity. A good leader can be trusted.
- Integrity. A good leader has principles and lives by them.
- Poise. A good leader is not overbearing, but friendly and assured.
- Thoughtfulness. S/he is considerate and aware.
- Common sense. A good leader has good judgment based on reason.
- Altruism. A good leader lives by the Golden Rule.
- Initiative. S/he gets things started now!
  —AUTHOR UNKNOWN

Supervising the Work of Others

A supervisor, more than anything else, is a leader. The supervisor accomplishes tasks through other people so that the organization's goals can be achieved. The supervisor sets the tempo, guides people's efforts, provides inspiration, and sometimes nudges people along, while at other times exercises discipline and delivers constructive criticism. Supervision is a constant balancing act of trying to keep a positive team spirit alive in a department or work unit. Supervision means setting goals and guiding staff toward them.

Some supervisors appear to have natural leadership ability, but most supervisors have had to develop their leadership skills through experience and training. Generally there are two kinds of management philosophies: authoritarian and participative (McGregor, 1960). Authoritarian management involves rigidly defined individual responsibility as a means of avoiding confusion as to who does what. It tends to foster competition among the members of a work unit. Generally, authoritarian management involves the assumption that people are passive, lack ambition, are indifferent to organizational needs, and need to be controlled. Authoritarian supervisors believe that their essential tasks are to direct, control, and motivate others.

Participative supervisors understand that their responsibility is flexible because it is clarified through discussion with subordinates and group consensus. Participative styles foster cooperation and teamwork among the members of a work unit. They are based on the assumption that people already have the motivation, the desire for development, and the readiness to direct their behavior to accomplish organizational goals. The essential tasks of participative supervisors are to arrange organizational conditions and methods of operation in such a way that people can achieve their own goals best by directing their efforts toward organizational objectives.

Not all that long ago most managers in this country believed in and practiced an authoritarian management style. But the authoritarian approach did not promote employee participation in the work process. The people performing the essential tasks of providing the services or producing the products were not involved in the workplace decisions that directly affected the quality of the services or products. Because of this, management and supervisors were uninformed about problems or opportunities for improvement, which then resulted in poor product quality and services.

After World War II, the Japanese adopted a philosophy of manufacturing quality control that was participative. It was important that they did this because their economy needed to be rebuilt after the war. They focused on continuous quality improvement and included employees in evaluating work processes, which enhanced product quality. As a result the Japanese have captured significant shares of markets, such as the automotive market, from U.S. manufacturers.

Since the mid twentieth century, more American managers have adopted the participative management style. They believe in the importance of ensuring that employee participation is built into work processes, so that quality products and services can be the outcome.

Some workplace decisions require quick decisiveness on the part of management where consensus and participation are not practical and should not be applied. Disasters and code blues are good examples of this in healthcare settings. In reality, most successful managers and supervisors know when to use participative leadership skills, when to use an authoritarian approach, or when to use a blend of both philosophies. There is a continuum of management styles, based on the urgency and complexity of the decision and level of employee expertise when making decisions.

To be effective, supervisors must have priorities on what to do. One of the most important tasks is that of teaching and training. When new people come on the job, it is the supervisor's responsibility to see to it that they know what they are doing before they are assigned a task to perform. If you as a supervisor simply assume that a new person can do the job, you may find yourself in lots of trouble.

Training responsibility involves more than instructing new staff. It is important for a supervisor to keep informed about new developments and information and pass that along to the staff. Whenever a new method of doing something or a new regulation is introduced, the supervisor must see to it that the staff has the skills necessary to perform those procedures.

Supervisors are also responsible for safety on the unit. Safety not only applies to all people in the facility, but to any equipment used as well. By setting a good example and applying the rules to everyone, the supervisor assures that the facility safety regulations are followed exactly.

Perhaps the most difficult responsibility of a supervisor is applying discipline. Authoritarian managers often use threats and abusive language to enforce discipline. This method is ineffective because it causes fear and resentment in staff, which slows down work and makes people uncooperative. A successful supervisor attempts to discipline using the positive approach. Positive discipline means that the person being disciplined should realize that the discipline is to help them do a better job and not to punish or embarrass them.

Positive discipline can be achieved by following these principles:

- Discipline should be handled professionally and impersonally, not as an attack on the individual.
- Discipline should be applied as soon as the situation will allow (but not when the supervisor is angry).
- Discipline should always apply to everyone in the same way.
- Staff members must be informed of rules and regulations in advance.

Both constructive criticism and discipline should be handled privately and confidentially. Certain exceptions apply if the facility is unionized and union representatives must be involved. Handling discipline on an impersonal basis means that the

Six Unforgivable Supervisory Mistakes

1. Treating individuals unequally because of sex, culture, age, disability, etc., which is illegal. Every employee deserves the same consideration.
2. Not keeping your word. The fastest way to destroy a trusting relationship with a subordinate is to make a promise and then break it.
3. Blowing hot and cold. Consistency is essential when managing. If you are positive one day and negative the next, staff will not know how to react. Respect for you will disappear.
4. Failure to follow basic company/facility policies and procedures. As a supervisor, you must handle your relationship with each staff member in a consistent and legal manner. This means doing things like documenting expectations and employee-improvement plans before telling your manager you wish to terminate an employee.
5. Losing your cool in front of staff. Everyone reaches a threshold of tolerance on occasion, but you need to keep your temper in check and your emotions under control. Blowing up can destroy relationships.
6. Engaging in a personal relationship with someone you supervise. No matter how close you are to staff members when you are both staff, when you are a supervisor, you change your role. It is poor practice to be in charge of a person during the day and personally involved with that individual after work.

discipline is directed against a behavior or violation, not against the person. A person is not punished because he or she failed to follow a safety regulation. The person is shown the serious consequences that could result from not complying with a rule designed to make the job (and the patient) safer.

It is also important for a supervisor to have a positive attitude. This is frequently not emphasized in training, but it is crucial for success. When a supervisor is positive, productivity improves. When a supervisor is negative, productivity drops. The challenge is to remain positive, even if those around you are not (see Table 6-1).

People are all motivated by essentially the same things. The desire for accomplishments, recognition, new challenges, and learning new things is the same for all people. Supervisors should strive to create an environment that fosters employee achievement and self-motivation.

TABLE 6-1   Successful/Unsuccessful Supervisory Traits

Successful Supervisor	*Unsuccessful Supervisor*
Remain positive under stress	Allow problems to get to you
Take time to teach what you know	Rush instructions to staff, then fail to follow up
Build/maintain rewarding relationships with subordinates	Be insensitive to subordinates' needs
Learn to set reasonable and consistent lines of authority	Be not interested in learning supervisory skills
Learn to delegate	Fail to understand that it isn't what a supervisor can do, but what he or she can get others to do
Establish standards of high quality and set good examples	Let your status go to your head
Work hard to become a good communicator	Offer one-way communication
Build team efforts to achieve high productivity	Become too authoritarian or too lax

As a supervisor, your responsibility is to manage your part of the overall business efficiently. You are responsible for the proper use of people, equipment, and resources. Efficient use of people, equipment, and supplies means making sure these resources are not wasted. Your efforts to get the job done correctly, efficiently, and on time are essential to the success of the facility.

Your relationship with patients is also very important in maintaining their satisfaction with the facility and care. If there is a delay, explain what is happening. If the patient has specific expectations about care, do your best to see that they are met, without violating facility policies, regulations, or safety standards. A good supervisor is also a salesperson selling the healthcare facility to patients. Many times a supervisor and staff do a great technical job with care but offend a patient in the process. The result is that the facility loses future business. On the other hand, if care goes poorly, a good supervisor who relates well with patients can still project a good facility image. Good customer relations are important because they develop goodwill and contribute to the growth of the facility.

Another responsibility you have as a supervisor is to your staff. You need to make sure that each person is working in a job s/he is best suited to handle. Training and

Effective supervision includes:

- being organized so that more time is available for goal-setting and dealing with subordinates.
- delegating effectively.
- communicating effectively.
- disciplining appropriately.

Supervisors who delegate effectively:

- explain importance of job.
- explain end results and let the employee determine how the task will be completed.
- clearly define the employee's authority and/or parameters that the employee has when completing the task.
- agree on a deadline and time frame with the employee.
- ask for feedback to ensure the employee completely understands the tasks and your expectations.
- provide controls to ensure the employee is on the right track.
- follow up and check on the employee's progress on a task.

education can help each person become better qualified and more productive. You are responsible for assigning daily tasks so that staff members on your team know what they are expected to do and when and how they are expected to do it.

You must ensure that each person has the necessary tools, equipment, and materials to safely complete their assigned job tasks. As a supervisor, you relay company policy to your staff. You have an obligation to present management directives to your staff as if they were your own. This is true even if you do not always completely agree with them. You are the link between your staff members and upper management. Successful supervisors can quickly gain respect and confidence by showing they will present their opinions to upper management and stand by them.

Successful supervisors know their people and realize that they have individual differences. You can learn about each person as an individual by listening and observing actions. You must be a problem-solver and let staff know they can come to you with their concerns. Be aware that staff members have personal problems away from the job that may affect their performance. In your supervisory role, you must be alert to these problems and be willing to help resolve them, along with job-related problems.

Supervisors need to create an organizational climate that motivates employees to perform their jobs effectively. They also need to look at their own behavior to ensure that employees feel respected and valued as members of the work team.

What Skills Are Required for a Charge Nurse?

Most healthcare facilities have a nurse in charge of each unit or shift. Most often they are called charge nurses. Some other names for the position are resource nurse or shift supervisor. Whatever the title, the role includes direct accountability for one unit during one shift. This is the first step in becoming a supervisor and usually a step before becoming a manager.

Outstanding charge nurses are easy to spot. They:

- support a successful quality-improvement program.
- achieve JCAHO accreditation with no contingencies.
- control total labor cost per patient day.
- control contract labor, such as registry/travelers, per patient day.
- achieve outstanding physician satisfaction survey results.
- achieve outstanding patient satisfaction survey results.
- support new-program implementation.
- maintain costs per unit within 5% of budget.

The charge nurses of the past were different than those needed today. The old model of charge nurse included difficult ideas such as, "The world is fair," or "There is a shortage and that's it." Charge nurses acted as if contract labor (registry and travelers) was inevitable, and that an all-RN model is best for patient care, even if it isn't practical in today's environment. Nursing salaries were perceived as pitifully poor and therefore it was assumed productivity could not be enhanced. It was assumed that all nurses were professionally motivated and would do things just because they needed doing. This mentality no longer has a place in health care.

The new charge nurse model is based on delivering quality and effective care at lower costs; using staff in differentiated roles based on education and training; working in a team model; focusing on high levels of patient, physician, and family

Supervisors who communicate effectively:

- plan for the communication with the employee by scheduling a time and planning what they want to say.
- are honest, candid, specific, factual and provide examples.
- open up communication with open-ended questions and remember to listen for two-way communication.
- ask for feedback to ensure that they and the employees have a shared understanding of the goal and to make the employees feel important enough to be asked for their views.

Supervisors that discipline appropriately:

- give facts and figures.
- help the employee understand why s/he is being disciplined, and define the problem.
- get agreement that a problem exists.
- look for solutions to resolve the performance problem/ conduct.

satisfaction; eliminating things nurses do that don't make a difference; being creative and innovative when solving problems; managing limited resources; and adopting a customer-focused orientation about nursing care.

Successful charge nurses now need to focus on using less management staff to support their decisions, identifying who is the coordinator of care (staff nurses), eliminating duplication, cross-training whenever possible, eliminating barriers between departments, and eliminating nonproductive time. They also set standards for quality and customer-service measures, rewards, and sanctions. Charge nurses help with making recruitment/retention, education, QA, UR, infection control, and risk management every unit's responsibility. Charge nurses made increased use of technology, staff by acuity as well as cost per unit of service, become more customer-sensitive, and streamline documentation.

For Your Toolkit

Lack of communication by nurse managers is a key reason for conflict with staff members.

Good communication skills are vital to developing a happy, productive staff willing to do more when crises arise. Because nurse managers often move between multiple units and balance their time between each unit, the charge nurse becomes the spokesperson for the nurse manager. This helps maintain patient care quality and satisfaction. Charge nurses manage day-to-day operations on a specific unit; the nurse manager oversees operations, and assures quality patient care, patient safety, staff development and education, staff satisfaction, recruitment, retention, financial analysis, and multidisciplinary meetings and teams.

The charge nurse becomes a crucial conduit for the nurse manager to staff on a unit. Open communication and candid conversations go a long way to preventing unresolved conflict. If there is an issue, talking about it is essential. Listening responsively to other individuals in the healthcare setting is also important, and charge nurses can provide that conduit as well. This creates mutual respect and collaboration, which improves both patient care and staff morale. Charge nurses are essential ingredients to making communication happen effectively on a unit.

For Your Toolkit

> **Being a nurse manager is the most challenging role in nursing.**

Mentoring and support for new charge nurses as well as resources and training are crucial to their success. Charge nurses need to be selected for their ability to supervise the work of others, as well as because they are good clinicians. Charge nurses support their nurse manager with key functions. The nurse manager role is probably the most difficult role in nursing. As a nurse manager, I always felt like I was stuck between the staff and nursing administration. I had 24-hour accountability, and without my charge nurses, I could never have made it work.

Key experience and attributes of a charge nurse in today's healthcare industry include*:

1. Education/experience
    *   RN license
    *   Three to four years experience as a staff RN with shift/team accountability
    *   Bachelor's degree completed or in progress

2. Technical expertise
    *   Understanding JCAHO accreditation and regulatory requirements
    *   Understanding of cost per unit standards
    *   Staff supervision and oversight
    *   Strong ability to plan and coordinate staff and unit activity

3. Basic skills
    *   Leadership
    *   Delegating
    *   Directing
    *   Motivating
    *   Supervising the work of others
    *   Organizational skills
    *   Critical-thinking skills
    *   Sound judgment

*Adapted from "Traits of an Indispensable Nurse," lecture by Richard Brock, RN, MN.

4. Decision-making ability

5. Integrity

6. Objective perspective/independent thinker

7. Strong work ethic/high energy level

8. Good time-management skills

9. Strong and positive self-image

10. Effective interpersonal skills

11. Flexible/adaptable and excited by change

12. Assertiveness and tenacity

13. Drive and personal ambition

14. Self-motivated/self-starter
    A competency profile for an outstanding charge nurse includes:
    Achievement competencies:
    *   Drive for achievement
    *   Initiative
    *   Concern for order
    Influence competencies:
    *   Interpersonal sensitivity
    *   Awareness and concern of personal impact
    *   Direct persuasion
    *   Use of influence strategies
    *   Organizational awareness
    *   Relationship building
    Self-management competencies:
    *   Self-confidence
    *   Tenacity
    *   Self-control
    *   Flexibility
    Problem-solving competencies:
    *   Use of concepts
    *   Analytical thinking
    *   Pattern recognition
    *   Technical expertise
    Managerial competencies:
    *   Development of others

- Directing others
- Management of groups
- Efficiency orientation
- Motivation of others
- Cause/effect thinking
- Creativity and innovation
- Calculated risk-taking
- Concern with image and impact
- Empathy

Knowledge/qualifications:

- Bachelor's degree
- Business appreciation

Social/communication skills:

- Fluent verbal skills
- Good listening skills
- Developing presentation skills
- Developing negotiation skills
- Positive self-presentation
- Rapport-building
- Social deportment
- Cooperativeness
- Ability to inspire others

Personal traits:

- Enthusiasm
- Decisiveness
- Stress tolerance
- Self-motivation
- Tolerance for ambiguity

Analyze your leadership strengths and weaknesses. Several leadership theories have been outlined in the business world over the past several decades. (See Table 6-2.)

TABLE 6-2 Leadership Theories

Theory	Driving Thought
Theory X	No one really wants to work
Theory Y	Individuals really want to make a contribution
Theory Z	People work best in teams
Theory C	If you satisfy the customer, you will have a future
Transformational leadership theory	Visionary, risk-taker, confidence builder, and change artist

In their book, the Komisarjevskys (2004) detail how being a good manager, or demonstrating your capability to be a good manager, requires many of the same skills as being a good parent.

Some say that leaders are born, not made. William A. Cohen (2004), PhD and retired major general of the U.S. Air Force, would beg to differ. "Leadership can be learned," he says. "It's a matter of not only having the qualities [of a leader], but knowing what to do" (Gates & Rubano, 2004). Even if you're a long shot for a promotion at work, ask the bosses to consider you—it will show you're ambitious and anxious for more responsibility. Or suggest creating a task force to temporarily fill the void left by the open position. Your boss will not only be impressed by your ambition but by your desire to lead as well.

The differences between managers and leaders are listed in Table 6-3.

Leaders are to professional nurses like yeast is to bread or fuel is to a rocket. You can't have one without the other. Managers and charge nurses need subordinates more

TABLE 6-3   Differences Between Managers and Leaders

Managers	Leaders
Do things right	Do the right things
Solve problems	Avoid problems
Follow direction	Obtain results
Manage productivity	Increase profits
Are efficient	Are effective
Maintain compliance	Improve the system
Control	Influence
Work in hierarchy	Work in networks
Make plans	Enhance learning
Create transaction	Create transformation
Administer	Innovate
Copy	Start from original
Maintain	Develop
Focus on systems and structure	Focus on people
Rely on control	Inspire trust
Use short-range viewpoint	Use long-range perspective
Keep eyes on bottom line	Have eyes on the horizon
Ask how and when	Ask what and why
Accept the status quo	Challenge status quo
Are classic good soldiers	Are individual persons

than subordinates need them. Managers get paid for what the subordinates do and create—not only for what they do themselves.

For Your Toolkit

> **Leaders are to professional nurses like yeast is to bread or fuel is to a rocket. You can't have one without the other.**

Charge nurses need to have:

- supervisory skills.
- the ability to respond to ambiguity and rapid change.
- the ability to manage self as well as others.
- the ability to communicate the organization's vision to employees.
- excellent time-management skills.
- the ability to be a positive, professional role model.
- the ability to develop trust in employees.
- the ability to foster innovation in employees.
- the ability to maintain perspective and sense of humor.

Charge nurse core competencies include:

- problem-solving ability.
- management skill.
- influence.
- social and communication skills.
- achievement.
- self-management.
- external focus.
- promoting vision and values for the future.
- promoting continual quality and process improvement.
- acting as a change agent.
- valuing people.
- demonstrating skills of management especially under circumstances of uncertainty or conflict.
- decentralizing information and authority.
- pursuing self-development.

Should You Be a Nurse Manager?

Managers are paid to make tough decisions. They must make trade-offs in how resources are distributed, balance different interests in complex and ambiguous situations, and use their influence to define their unit's interests without undermining the performance of the entire organization (Hill, 1998). Managers need power to do this type of work, but power does not come from formal authority. What is required to do the job well is not just being in control, but gaining the support and commitment of subordinates, peers, and higher-ups as collaborators. Formal authority can often affect changes in behavior, but for commitment or changes in attitude, managers have to share their power.

For Your Toolkit

> **Sharing power with others actually increases a manager's influence.**

The idea of empowerment makes one think of losing control; however, sharing power with others actually increases a manager's influence in a situation. This is the paradox of power. Empowerment means sharing the potential to influence others. By granting others the autonomy to do their jobs, and sharing information and expertise to ensure they make sound judgment calls, managers can have great influence over workers. The manager still sets the agenda within which work should be accomplished, but those closest to the action can figure out tactics and solve problems.

It gets a bit stickier when a manager must influence those over whom s/he has no direct or formal authority. In order to influence folks over whom you have no authority, you need allies. Peers as well as higher-ups are sources of critical information, resources, and collaboration. By setting up a network with these folks, a manager creates allies. When a manager creates allies, s/he enhances his or her influence as well as the ability to get the job done.

Smart managers regard anyone they depend on as a potential ally, even if the individual appears to be an adversary. The focus is on building mutually beneficial alliances by discerning what the manager can offer that others may need or want. In order to exercise influence through exchange, you must first identify those on whom you depend, and then step into their shoes to see the world from their perspective. In order to use this strategy, you must know whom you depend on and why, whose cooperation and compliance is needed, and whose opposition will keep you from accomplishing your work. Your source of power becomes what you have to offer that they need or want, and what they have to offer that you need or want. Trust drives your ability to create power. Mutual trust will allow you to build influence.

When assessing relationships and making sense of situations in which there are perceived conflicts of interest, it is likely that managers determine their own behavior as honorable, and that of other persons as self-aggrandizing, irrational, or ambitious. It is important not to attribute malicious motives to those opposing you in a conflict situation. It is important for you to test your assumptions and adopt a broader perspective—this is crucial for win-win negotiations.

Ensuring you have a network that includes relationships with many different people is hard work but worthwhile. It is how you can be successful as a manager. Because most of us are most comfortable with people similar to us, the larger challenge lies in bridging differences. Concentrate on people who are critical to success but with whom you do not necessarily have a well-developed relationship.

Trust is a function of how an individual perceives a manager in three areas: competence (does s/he know the right thing to do?), character (does s/he want to do the right thing?), and influence (can s/he get it done?). The more trust people have in you, the less often they will require proof that you will deliver what you have promised. This kind of flexibility is invaluable to managers, especially during organizational upheavals.

Thinking about influence as an exchange can lead some managers to be exploitative. Remember, to work, networks have to be mutually beneficial. Treating people fairly is to treat them on the basis of what *they* need. Exercising influence depends on being clear about that concept. Be aware of not only achieving your immediate objective, but also how your actions will affect a relationship over time. Influence is about building interdependencies, and creating partnerships is one of the most rewarding aspects of management. (See Table 6-4.)

TABLE 6-4   Responsibilities of Managers in Leadership Roles

Be the source of a vision

Establish and maintain trust

Serve as a political conduit

Serve as ethical standard bearer for the unit/department

Make decisions

Make effective and appropriate judgments

Expand awareness of staff

Become a spark

Build a framework for effective communication

Adopt a constant planning perspective and attitude

Being a nurse manager can be one of the most rewarding career moves a nurse can make. It can also be the most frustrating. Being a manager involves being a leader as well as supervising the work of others. You are both the drum major leading the parade and the band master pushing from the rear of the band to keep things moving. I have been in about eight different types of management roles in my career. I have learned much about how to manage in 30 years in nursing—both from doing it right *and* doing it wrong. If you are considering moving into nursing management, there are some issues you need to evaluate.

Are you willing to get additional training? Expanding your job-related education is an effective way to move ahead. Obtaining an academic degree isn't always necessary, but acquiring essential management skills definitely is. Employers are looking for excellent written and oral communication skills and an ability to effectively manage staff and workloads. If you are interested in a promotion to management, consider taking classes that focus on supervision and communication skills. There are national programs that offer one-day seminars and local college and online course options.

Are you able to coach others? The ability to motivate others and oversee their work is critical in all nursing roles, but particularly in management. If you are a computer whiz, offer to train co-workers, even if it is not part of your present job description. This will provide supervisory experience beyond the scope of your job. Whenever possible, volunteer to oversee *per diem* or registry staff, or head up a committee or project. These activities will help you learn how to give clear directions and tactfully to check to see that the work is progressing correctly and in a timely manner. Evaluate your awareness that there are multiple ways to get a job done effectively and a job can be well done—even if it isn't done the way you would do it. (The art of coaching is discussed in depth in Chapter 7 on coaching/mentoring.)

Can you make decisions and delegate? Both are key functions of managers. If you are a parent or care for a dependent, you likely already do both well. Managers must assign tasks, plan projects, and make numerous choices daily. Practice these skills on your job, at home, or in community activities. Become active in professional nursing organizations and take on leadership roles. Learn how to give assignments to others, taking care to provide the time and resources necessary to help them complete the tasks at hand.

Do you have the initiative and willingness to take on responsibility? Managers must be able to operate independently and be self-directed. They must be able to make significant contributions to productivity and the financial bottom line of a facility. With more regulations, shorter lengths of stay, and higher patient acuity, managers have to work faster and smarter just to stay up with the workload. Make it a habit to ask for more work and expand the scope of your current job. This will help you get used to the frequent requests from your boss to "take a look at this situation and give me your recommendations" that come with being a manager. Contribute new ideas to management for ways to improve your department or unit.

Do you have strong communication skills? The ability to listen, explain clearly, and give precise directions is crucial. Oral and written communication skills are paramount for management success, but communicating effectively also means using technology to transmit information. Practice speaking at and facilitating meetings. Volunteer to serve on department committees and be an active participant. Improve your written skills by writing reports or correspondence.

Are you a good listener? Listening is a critical part of communication and is covered in Chapter 4 on communication skills. Employers want managers who ask for and listen to ideas and suggestions. Pay close attention as colleagues state their requests or outline a problem. Be conscious of letting a person explain while you take in what is being said. Do not interrupt. Managers, however hurried or pressured they may be, need to allow others to express themselves completely, whenever possible. Once you have heard everything, formulate your response. This way, both employers and those you supervise will view interactions with you in a positive way.

Have you studied other managers? Observe managers you respect and those you don't respect and analyze their skills. How assertive are they? How do they make decisions? Are they polite and respectful of employees and subordinates? Do they listen? Do they accept feedback graciously? Do they follow up with employee issues? Emulate their strengths to develop your own style. Learn how to handle problems by watching what managers do well or not so well.

You can also learn a lot by watching someone who is an ineffective manager. Learning how *not* to behave can be as valuable as following a positive role model. Seek advice on how to motivate others and manage workload. People work hardest for and are most loyal to managers who praise and reward good work.

Do you use professional ethics? Managers must display high moral standards. Do you respect other employees? Are you careful not to offend other staff? Are you sensitive to diversity issues? Are you careful not to use terminology that others might deem offensive? Do you treat all people fairly? In today's healthcare environment, it is especially important to show a high level of integrity and avoid actions that could be seen as discriminatory or harassing or that demonstrate a different care standard for different patients.

Can you handle deadlines as well as set and meet goals? The higher in an organization you move, the more pressure you will encounter, so you need to develop coping mechanisms that will help you handle challenges without burning out. Good time-management skills and organizing your work efficiently are essential. When you plan projects, develop a time line that outlines the tasks. As your workload and the number of staff under you increase, you will need to become extremely well organized. You need to create a foundation to deal effectively with problems as they arise.

Another essential skill for leadership is observation. Notice who the leaders are. True leaders are individuals to whom people gravitate. Using a true leader as a model offers valuable insight into your own behavior, as well as an expert with whom you can discuss what works and what doesn't. Keep in mind that not all modeling experiences are positive. I have learned a lot about how *not* to behave by watching some leaders in nursing.

Leaders actually lead by using effective communication, empowering followers, having a clear vision, seeing the bigger picture, navigating around potential pitfalls, and having positive self-confidence. Leaders tend to fail when success goes to their heads, they establish a personal kingdom, and they mislead themselves into believing they are infallible and need no one else. One way to keep your ego in check as a leader is to realize that leaders wouldn't have a role to lead without people to lead. Therefore, a crucial duty is to empower your followers by creating a sense of significance, competence, and community. Keeping open lines of honest communication and showing employees how their work contributes to a meaningful end is a great way to create an all-inclusive environment for success.

When evaluating your potential as a manager, there are a few areas to consider, such as decision-making strategies, problem-solving skills, self-confidence, interpersonal skills, facilitation, adaptability, integrity, commitment, and empathy. Assessing your own strengths and weaknesses will allow you to see where your skills are developmentally at the present time. This requires honesty about the raw materials you have to work with. Evaluating where you are will help you determine what you hope to become as a manager. Can you do all the things just listed? Then a management role could be next up for you.

Now that you are willing to consider a management position, there are some additional things you need to know. First and foremost, if you are going to lead, lead well. There are plenty of lousy nurse managers. We don't need more. We have all worked with toxic managers, and it is extremely demoralizing. Effective, positive managers are also linked to staff retention. All the best recruitment strategies are for naught if staff members leave because of a toxic manager.

As a new manager, you will want to create a few strategies to enhance your chance of success. Here are some strategies I have used effectively when starting in a new management role.

- Open your office door and be available and visible. Staff members aren't sure what you are up to if they can't see you.
- Be seen. Hanging out with staff at planned meetings, lunches, and breaks works very well. You can learn more about what is happening on your unit by hanging around the coffee pot than you ever will in a meeting.

- Be honest and deal with staff fears like system changes, reductions in force, or staff shortages. Staff may not talk about what they are really worried about when you are new, so you need to talk about what you think people are really thinking and feeling. When fears are mentioned out in the open and discussed, you can create trust and establish a relationship.

Don't fall into the common trap of assuming people will know how to act if you are their manager. Many managers assume that subordinates will read their minds to understand what the manager wants in terms of outcomes and behavior. Some managers believe that if people are smart enough, they will just figure out what they want. Nothing is further from the truth. Staff members need to be clear on your expectations and understand your style. It's great if employees can read the subtle nuances in your behavior and figure out exactly what you require of them, but most people aren't mind readers. Even those who are smart may be oblivious to what's important to you unless you spell it out.

If the CEO of the hospital visits your department, some of your employees will naturally put a best foot forward and do a good job of demonstrating that "everything is fine here!" but many will use the opportunity to reveal problems and frustrations. If you want those employees to behave differently, you will need to explain how you want them to behave when a top administrator comes on the unit.

In most hospital departments, employees asking for information get it, but most managers prefer that certain kinds of information be withheld or glossed over with a VIP on the unit. It may seem that you really should not have to ask people to do what they have to do to make the department, the hospital, them—and you—look good. It's not that these things are immoral. It's just that they lie outside of what we consider usual job requirements. People are often given incomplete or incorrect information and are expected to know exactly what to use and what to disregard. Twenty percent of your staff will know. The other 80% will be confused, frustrated, and ultimately inefficient.

Counting on employees to read minds is an all-too-common management style that often results in disappointment and distrust. Managers are impatient and irritated with employees who need more specific information. Employees sense that they have disappointed the boss but usually have no idea what they need to do to meet expectations. After all, they are not mind readers.

All skills and abilities are distributed along a normal curve. This means that 20% of any group will be superior performers, 60% will be average, and 20% below average (Bernstein and Craft-Rozen, 1995). Some folks are at the top end of the normal curve for observational learning. This is the learning people do by watching successful people and imitating what they do.

Studies show that about 20% of any group of employees will be good enough at learning by observation to figure out what it is expected (Bernstein and Craft-Rozen, 1995). These employees need minimal direction and little support. Bosses often see these top performers and wonder why the rest of their employees can't figure out what it takes. They expect the same behaviors and abilities from the other 80% and both sides end up frustrated.

Intelligent people often assume that everybody else knows as much as they know and can do what they do. They might think of people who can't do what they do as stupid, but more often they will see them as lacking motivation. When we know something, it seems so obvious that we forget how it felt not to know it. To others, however, who don't know exactly what we know in the way that we know it, we appear to expect them to be mind readers. The illusion is that getting better at our jobs means building up an ever-enlarging collection of facts. The facts come early in the learning process. Increases in skill don't come from an increase in the store of facts in your head, but rather in the ability to make finer and finer distinctions.

Most managers may be good at doing but may not be skilled at analyzing what they do and explaining it to other people. They may also assume that explaining is what teachers do. In reality, the best managers have the skills of good teachers. Teachers assume that students don't know what the teacher knows and that the main purpose of teaching is to get them to understand the subject as well as the teacher does. Too many managers think that employees already know whatever they need to know. Nothing is further from the truth.

One of the real tests of your skill as a manager is the effect you have on the majority of people who don't intuitively know what you want. These people are paying attention to some cues, but those cues may not be the ones you want them to follow. The more you manage, the more effective you will be and the less mind-reading will be required.

Decide what you want your staff to know. Before you teach them, understand exactly what you want your staff to learn. Let them know in advance what they are supposed to do, when to do it, and how they can meet your expectations. Ask for what you want and don't assume that people know what to do. Most people know the basics of the job. What you need them to learn specifically are matters of style and the manner in which things are done on your unit. They must also understand and be sensitive to the political realities in your facility. It's probably best to assume that the people you manage know absolutely nothing about these kinds of things except what you tell them. Set priorities and tell people what they are. Break complex skills into parts when you explain them. Use examples that apply to your unit. Encourage questions as you teach.

For Your Toolkit

Reward good work, and that behavior will happen more often.

Reward good work and it will happen more often. Usually the strategy of managers is to do the opposite. As long as employees are doing what they are supposed to be doing, they are ignored. Then, when they step out of line, they are punished. Punishing negative behavior is much less effective than rewarding positive behavior. The more payoff there is for doing what you want, the more likely you are to get it.

It is difficult to instill attitudes that lead to correct behavior. Make a practical, detailed request and even show people what you want if you can. Tell them why they should do it. You don't need to worry what they are thinking while they are doing what you want. That will come with time, as they gain experience.

You will also need to talk to your employees. Ask about and listen to their concerns. Ask questions to determine their understanding of how things really are. The better you know them, the better you will know what they need to know. Short, regular meetings for exactly this purpose are helpful. The more you can get your employees to talk to you, the more effective you can be as their boss.

You will also need to tell them explicitly what is to be done in certain situations. Tell it like it is, even if you are embarrassed. Give them examples of what is appropriate or inappropriate, even if the examples are difficult or embarrassing for you. You will be much more embarrassed if the people you oversee don't know these things.

Be sure you deal with conflict. Groups of people and team members invariably experience conflict. Many managers choose to ignore conflict when new to a role and hope that it will go away. Some choose to use coercion to get staff to change. As many of us have experienced, this doesn't work well. To deal with conflict among your staff, start by asking those who disagree to paraphrase one another's comments. This may help them learn whether they really understand each other. Work out a compromise. Agree on the underlying source of conflict and then engage in give-and-take discussions to agree on a solution. Ask each person to list what the others should do. Exchange lists and select a compromise that all are willing to accept—even if they don't like it.

You may need to convince some team members that they have to admit they were incorrect. Help them save face by convincing them that changing a position may actually show strength and maturity. Last but not least, respect the experts on your team. Give their opinions more weight when the conflict involves their expertise, but don't rule out conflicting opinions. Creative conflict resolution can be positive for everyone involved.

Be sure you share information. Staff need to know what upper management is thinking and planning. If staff feel uninformed, they perceive changes are being "done to them" instead of feeling they are involved in making the changes. Use newsletters, email memos, and regular meetings to keep staff up to date. Involve your employees. Ask staff for input and ideas on how to improve services or enhance systems. Reward innovators and follow up on suggestions.

Remember to give yourself time. It takes time for new managers to learn how to be effective. It takes time for staff to trust and respect new managers. Be patient, and remember that you cannot rush the process of learning how to be a good manager. Research studies identify retention strategies related to the work environment as critical to employee satisfaction. Fifty percent of employee satisfaction comes from the relationship with bosses (Kaye and Jordan-Evan, 2002). Research shows that the quality of the relationship between a boss and subordinate is a primary predictor of an employee's intention to remain in a current workplace.

An investment in strengthening an organization's leaders—from senior executives to middle managers to team leaders—pays off in all sorts of ways, but particularly in attracting and retaining employees. Nurse managers have a responsibility to learn how to manage proactively and effectively. This benefits not only their individual lifelong learning, but their employees' well-being and satisfaction with the organization.

Those hospitals that have measures in place to hold managers accountable for retention tend to experience lower turnover rates. Accountability measures can include incorporation of retention efforts into the managers' performance appraisal process, bonuses for taking action related to turnover or achieving a qualitative or quantitative change in the turnover rate, and periodic review of employee satisfaction in the manager's specific service area (Abrams, 2002). (See Table 6-5.)

Focusing on retention strategies means facilities cannot ignore the effect that leadership style has on retention. Toxic nurse executives and middle managers can sabotage retention efforts by driving away nurses at all levels of the organization. The best retention strategies in the world will not work if retention is inhibited by self-centered, power-hungry leaders.

Hospitals and nursing staff both are wary of nurse executives and managers who impede retention by setting up a personal kingdom instead of working with others as

TABLE 6-5   Managerial Risk and Rewards

Risks of Being a Manager	Rewards of Being a Manager
Inability to be positive 100% of time	Empowerment
Increased stress	Increased self-confidence
Lack of security	Expanding horizons
Feel caught in the middle	Personal growth
Crises-oriented basis of function	Satisfaction from helping others grow
Changing relationships	Building professionalism/pride
Failure	Success
Doesn't feel fun anymore	Feel passionate and excited about work

a team, use fear and intimidation to get tasks completed, have a "my way or the high-way" mentality, make negative comments about staff, or blame subordinates for decisions that result in poor outcomes. Nursing staff who work under retention-inhibiting conditions often complain about their work environment and change jobs. Toxic attitudes can spread outward and cause a ripple effect that can damage an entire facility and take years to repair.

For Your Toolkit

A positive leadership style is a cornerstone of success as well as a key retention strategy.

A positive leadership style is a cornerstone of success as well as a key retention strategy. Nurse leaders who reward efforts with positive feedback, encouragement, and coaching are also retaining staff. Career enhancement as well as retention-focused behaviors include empowerment of staff at all levels, coaching for both positive change and to eliminate negative behaviors, choosing to mentor both new nurses and new managers, investment in training and skill-building for all levels of staff, implementing change with a teamwork-based model, encouraging innovation and out-of-the-box thinking for care management and work redesign changes, and proactive planning instead of reactivity.

Some additional management thoughts include:

- **Never forget what it's like to be in the trenches**. My first job was as a nurses' aide on evening shift in a skilled nursing home. I never want to forget the difference between feelings I had having a charge nurse say "thank you" or get angry at me for not be able to follow through on a task. I want to be sure I remember to manage others the way I would like to be managed.
- **Graciousness and common courtesy go a long way.** "Please," "thank you," and "I appreciate you working an extra shift" are not used nearly enough by nurse managers. It takes two seconds to say please or thank you and the payback is endless. It also builds staff loyalty and willingness to help you achieve departmental goals.
- **Build trust.** Trust is a critical element to build with employees. It is also something that is earned, not given freely by employees and subordinates. When employees trust their manager, they will do anything to help accomplish goals and objectives.
- **Relationship management matters.** Most nurses hate politics and consider management roles to be very political. The reality is that management is all about

managing relationships. You need to build strong allies in key departments to help you manage your work. Managing relationships builds trust as well as gives you individuals to network with to get the job done. Consider managing relationships to be the most important thing you do as a manager.

- **Being a good manager is not the same as being popular.** Many decisions you make as a manager will be difficult and make at least some staff unhappy. You will need to learn to accept that making the right decision for your unit doesn't always make you popular with your staff.

- **Never ask someone to do something you wouldn't do yourself.** Employees need to know that you understand what it is like to be in the trenches. If you ask an employee to pick up trash, be sure you are willing to do it yourself before you ask. If you ask staff members to do only the things that you don't like to do, they will recognize it and be resentful and unwilling to help. Staff will watch to see if you live up to what you ask of others.

- **If you ask staff members their opinions, be prepared to do something with the answers.** It is crucial to get staff feedback on issues related to care of patients and department goals and objectives. Keep in mind that if you ask opinions, the expectation is that you do something with the answers. Don't ask the question if you already know how you want to proceed—you will alienate employees. If you do ask for input, then provide follow-up to staff about how it was used in the final decision-making process.

- **Manage by walking around.** This is a relatively old concept in business, but many nurse managers don't use it. You can learn more about what is happening with your staff and what is working or not working on your unit in 10 minutes of walking around than you can in a month of meetings. Get out of your office and talk to staff. You will be amazed at what you learn.

- **Delegate and then get out of the way.** Many nurse managers believe in delegation but can't actually let go of a process or project to let someone else take the reins. Meet with the staff to share the goal and outcome needed and provide the boundaries and any mandates that must be included. Give clear expectations and a completion date. Offer to be available for meetings and guidance. Then get out of the way and let the employees do their thing. Ask for feedback and follow-up. If they fail to deliver, you have learned a valuable lesson and so has the employee. More often than not, the staff member will deliver a successfully completed project and you will have time to spend on other issues.

- **Embrace and manage change**. Transition is a steady, constant state, according to Mitchell Marks (1994). Change never stops in health care; therefore, transition is always present. Learn to embrace it instead of fighting it. Learn about the change process and understand your feelings about each step. This will help you anticipate what may be your most difficult change when you encounter it. Embrace the change process with your staff as an opportunity to excel and achieve more that benefits patient care.

- **Be a risk-taker**. Many nurse managers are so worried about failure that they never take a chance on doing things differently. Failure is not a bad thing. Doing nothing means a missed opportunity. Learn to trust your intuition on how to proceed with new ideas, much as you have trusted it to tell you when a patient takes a turn for the worse. Some of the best things that have been implemented in health care happened because a nurse manager took the risk to try something new.

- **Strive to become a leader, not just a manager**. Several business gurus like Deming and Peter Drucker have identified the differences between management and leadership. One of the common threads in these business theories is that managers "do things right," but leaders "do the right things." Leaders are not always the most popular, but they are always respected.

- **Build bridges, not kingdoms**. One of the worst mistakes you can make as a nurse manager is to use your authority to build personal power. Nothing will cause you to be disrespected more quickly than forgetting that being a nurse manager is about being there for the staff members who work to support you—not just thinking of your own personal gain.

- **Being a good manager means empowerment.** As a manager you are not a problem-solver as when you were as a staff nurse. You need to get into the role of being a facilitator and a coach. Anyone can give advice, but it takes a good manager to empower employees to solve problems on their own.

- **Communicate often and tell the truth.** You may not always be able to share good news, but ongoing honest and effective communication is critical to your success. Tell the truth. Never say "never" and remember to be human. If you lead with your heart first, then your head, you will do well as a manager.

- **Use the 24-hour rule.** Never make a difficult decision right away if you can avoid doing so. Taking an extra 24 hours to make a decision may save you lots of trouble (or embarrassment) later.

- **Remember that people are like popcorn.** People learn differently and at different speeds. People "pop" at different times. Some of your staff will understand exactly what you want them to do the first time you explain it. Others will take longer. Be patient with those who "pop" slower than others. It doesn't mean they're resisting—they just may not get it yet. Continue to make your request and explain the rationale. There are very few dud employees. Eventually, most of them get it and are happy to help achieve departmental and organizational objectives.

- **Let go of vibrating poles.** There are multiple issues in healthcare organizations that can make you crazy. Our natural tendency as nurses is to try and control things so we can fix them. Most healthcare facilities are dysfunctional, and we can't change anything. As we continue to try to control whatever is dysfunctional,

Turner's Tips for Management Success

- *Never* forget what it's like to be in the trenches.
- Graciousness and common courtesy go a long way.
- Build trust.
- Relationship management matters.
- Being a good manager is not the same as being popular.
- Never ask someone to do something you wouldn't do yourself.
- If you ask staff members their opinions, be prepared to do something with the answers.
- Manage by walking around.
- Delegate and then get out of the way.
- Embrace and manage change.
- Be a risk-taker.
- Strive to become a leader, not just a manager.
- Build bridges, not kingdoms.
- Being a good manager means empowerment.
- Communicate often and tell the truth.
- Use the 24-hour rule.
- Remember that people are like popcorn.
- Let go of vibrating poles.
- Make sure you fight over only silver bullets.
- Remember that the patient is what matters the most.

the more frustrated we get, and still nothing changes. A healthcare organization is the equivalent of a vibrating pole. The temptation is to hang on to the pole to make it stop vibrating. In reality, that makes both you and the pole vibrate. The answer is to let go of the pole. Not easy to do in work settings, but it may be the only thing that will save your sanity.

- **Make sure you fight over only silver bullets.** There are many problems in healthcare organizations, and it is tempting to try and solve all of them. Choose fighting issues carefully. Not every issue is worth going to the mat over. Pick the

TABLE 6-6   Old Management Versus New Management

Old Way of Managing (Authoritarian)	*New Way of Managing (Participative)*
Rigidly defined individual responsibilities	Flexible definition of responsibilities of team members via discussion and consensus
Fosters competition between individuals	Fosters cooperation and teamwork among members
Assumes that staff are passive, lack ambition, and need controlling	Assumes that staff have motivation and readiness to direct behavior toward organizational goals
Management is to direct, control, and motivate others	Arrange organizational conditions and operations so staff can achieve their own goals best by directing efforts toward organization objectives
Quality is fine the way it is	Quality can and must improve
Checking data/reports ensures quality	Analysis and improving processes ensure quality
People cause defects and poor quality	Processes and systems cause defects and poor quality
Intuition and technology will solve problems	Collecting data and acting with knowledge will solve problems
Quality costs money	Quality saves money
Customers are problems	Customers are partners
Suppliers/vendors are problems	Suppliers/vendors are partners
We don't have time for quality and customer service	We don't have time not to have quality and customer service

issues that will make the most difference to patient care or that compromise your ethics or integrity. The rest probably don't matter that much. Ask yourself if this issue will make a difference in a year. If the answer is no, move on.

- **Remember that the patient is what matters the most.** It is easy to get lost in personnel, project, and budget/productivity issues. Try and remember that the reason you are a healthcare manager is to make a difference to the *patient*. Always keep patients' needs as your central priority—you will rarely be faulted for doing so.

Managing an Effective Team

The key to your success as a supervisor or manager is the relationship between you and your work group. You are dependent on your group and you need it as much as it needs you. Organizations use the concept of synergy: teams can accomplish much more than individual members can by working alone. Most facilities cannot accomplish goals without teamwork because the goals cannot be achieved by each supervisor or staff member individually.

Calling a group a team doesn't make it a team. When teamwork is appropriate and desirable, a formal team structure is not always necessary. Creating a team for the sake of having a team is a bad idea. Some nursing tasks require teamwork and others require individual effort. Teamwork is accomplished by making sure that cooperative behavior is positively reinforced.

In a team model of nursing care, the team works toward the goal of managing the patient's care as directed by the physician. All care is coordinated by the primary nurse or case manager and is done in conjunction with the patient and involved family members (Turner, 1998). The most effective healthcare work environment is one in which people know when to work alone and when to ask for help. When you need to work with others to develop a solution to a complex problem, teams produce effective resolutions.

For Your Toolkit

The key to your success as a supervisor or manager is the relationship between you and your work group.

Bringing teams together increases the opportunity for positive reinforcement among team members. Peers exert tremendous influence on behavior. If team members are taught how to reinforce one another positively for efforts made and results achieved, the outcome will be effective teamwork. Team members have more contact with one another than do their managers, so reinforcement can be more frequent, and because they are together while the work is occurring, reinforcement is likely to be immediate.

There are several essential elements that differentiate a team from a group of people. Within teams:

- group members must have shared goals or a reason for working together.
- group members must be interdependent on each others' experience, abilities, and commitment in order to achieve mutual goals.
- group members must be committed to the idea that working together leads to more effective decisions than working alone.
- group must be accountable as a functioning unit within a larger organizational context, such as a hospital (Robbins, 2002).

Making a group into a team means more, however, than assuring the presence of the four elements of shared goals, interdependencies, commitment, and accountability. The aim of team-building is to help a group evolve into a cohesive unit whose members not only share the same high expectations for accomplishing group tasks, but also trust and support one another and respect one another's individual differences. Teams that work together do well; teams with internal dissension don't work well.

Characteristics of Effective Team Members

Effective team members:

- support the team leader.
- help the team leader to succeed.
- ensure all viewpoints are explored.
- express opinions, both for and against an idea.
- compliment the team leader on team efforts.
- provide open, honest, and accurate information.
- act in a positive and constructive manner.
- provide appropriate feedback.
- understand personal and team roles.
- bring problems to the team.
- accept ownership for team decisions.
- recognize that they each serve as team leaders at certain times.
- balance appropriate levels of participation.
- participate voluntarily.
- maintain confidentiality.
- show loyalty to the company, team leader, and team.
- view criticism as an opportunity to learn.
- state problems, along with alternative solutions and options.
- give praise and recognition when warranted.
- operate within the boundaries of team rules.
- confront the team leader when his/her behavior is not helping the team.
- share ideas freely and enthusiastically.
- encourage others to express their ideas fully.
- ask one another for opinions and listen to them.
- criticize ideas, not people.
- avoid disruptive behavior such as side conversations and inside jokes.
- avoid defensiveness when fellow team members disagree with their ideas.
- attend meetings regularly, promptly, and enthusiastically.

Adapted from *Supervisory Training Modules,* Beverly Health and Rehab., adapted 2005.

Nursing care teams usually consist of RNs, LVN/LPNs, and CNAs. CNAs who work entirely on their own to the exclusion of other team members will create gaps in services and continuity of care. CNAs must work in collaboration with other teams and departments to promote quality services. This also happens when licensed nurses working on their own exclude the CNAs. This results in the same disruption of quality of care. Quality care and efficient service mean working together. If you are a supervisor, your task is to build a work group of willing, cooperative members who work together in a climate of acceptance, support, and trust. In short—a team.

Effective teams have high productivity and morale. They tend to develop their own social systems and high levels of group loyalty. Sometimes they develop elitist attitudes and see themselves as better than other groups.

Effective team members:

- understand and are committed to team goals.
- are friendly, concerned, and interested in others.
- acknowledge and confront conflict openly.
- listen to others with understanding.
- include others in the decision-making process.
- recognize and respect individual differences.
- contribute ideas and solutions.
- value and respect others' ideas and contributions.
- recognize and reward team efforts.
- encourage and appreciate feedback about team performance.

An effective team is one that can solve its own problems, and the ability to solve problems is predicated on the ability to identify and remove obstacles that deflect energy away from those problems. When team members expend energy on hidden agendas, internal conflicts, role ambiguity, or confusion about the team's mission or value, they cannot focus their best efforts on solving work-related problems. The process of team-building seeks to improve members' problem-solving abilities by enabling them to confront and manage issues that hinder their functioning as a unit.

Team-building does not happen quickly. It is an ongoing process, and the personality of the team will change as employees grow in their jobs, add to their capabilities, or as the team gains or loses members. As a team leader you can help ensure the effectiveness of your team by helping your team members recognize their strengths and abilities. Team members need to be encouraged to develop their individual skills and be given the opportunity to stretch those skills. In addition, supervisors should focus on specific actions.

Treat your team members as you would want them to treat patients. Make it clear that you expect them to treat one other with the same respect and level of service that they show their patients. Foster cooperation rather than competition among the members of

For Your Toolkit

Treat your team members as you would want them to treat patients.

your team. Be sure your team members know that no one stands alone. When they need support or a backup person, another team member should always be available.

Be supportive and available to your team members. Let them know they can come to you any time with questions, problems, suggestions, or ideas. Don't smother initiative, and get out of their way if they are doing a good job. Give suggestions, encouragement, support, and a sympathetic ear when it is needed.

Communication is the primary factor in developing teams. Teams are more than a group with a single goal. They are composed of individuals with unique talents and personalities. It takes time to build the level of trust needed among team members. It is communication that makes that a reality.

Understanding your group-member dynamics will make you a more effective supervisor. Observing your members and getting to know them is the key to understanding their individual contributions to the group. Understanding the interactions among members will help you when you need to choose people for a new project. Taking advantage of a team member's natural skills and talents will help the team reach its goals.

Most people want the chance to be a member of a winning and productive team. They want the opportunity to contribute. That basic desire will help you to build a great team. It takes patience, but it is worth the time and energy.

The supervisor is an important part of the total team system. Highly effective work groups see their supervisors as:

- supportive, friendly, and helpful.
- having confidence in the team's ability and integrity.
- having high performance expectations.
- providing necessary training and coaching.
- viewing errors as learning opportunities rather than opportunities to criticize.

Building a highly effective team starts with selecting and training qualified group members. The hiring process should include an interpersonal skills assessment of candidates to determine their abilities to work well with others in a team setting. Once they are hired, be sure they are thoroughly oriented to their job.

Allow the team members the opportunity to influence group goals and the freedom to contribute to those goals. This will allow you to concentrate on solving problems that interfere with goal achievement and on building a positive identity for the work team. This identity must end up as a collective ego of individuals. Self-interested individuals destroy teamwork. Each team member must be professional, know his/her role, and perform at the highest level. Supervisors must train each team member to allow each team member to provide necessary skills. The trust and loyalty of the group will develop over time as the team works together.

Supervisors must create team-building in four areas:

1. Providing support is crucial. These are things you do to increase or maintain each group member's sense of personal worth and importance as a team member such as providing encouragement and recognition for good performance, speaking out on behalf of group members, and referring others directly to group members to answer questions or solve problems.
2. Promoting interaction between members encourages relating. These are things you do to create or maintain a network of interpersonal relationships among group members, such as sponsoring or encouraging group social events, holding work group meetings, and arranging lunch breaks so that group members can be together.
3. Emphasizing group goals are the things you do to create a high level of awareness and commitment to deliver a product or service to your customers by creating, changing, clarifying, and gaining acceptance of group goals. This is typically done best through the involvement and participation of group members.
4. The last area supervisors must focus on is facilitating group task accomplishment. These are things you do to provide effective work methods, facilities, equipment, and schedules for accomplishing group goals. This includes solving problems that your group has with other groups it works with to achieve goals. Sometimes this involves resolving conflict between team members.

These four areas of development are essential for an effective team. However, the supervisor is not the only person who needs to contribute to the group in these areas. In highly effective groups, team members help each other. The supervisor's attitude and patterns of involvement tend to be mirrored in the behavior of the group members. Therefore, the responsibility for group success and effectiveness is placed on all members of the team.

Supervisors need to manage teams more as a coach than as a boss. This means that staff needs to understand in behavioral terms what they are to do. The team leader must clarify what group members are to do through coaching. (See Table 6-7.)

Changing behavior requires many reinforcements of the new behavior before new habits are successfully entrenched. You cannot reinforce a team. You can only reinforce team-member behavior. You can reward a team, but it works best when all members are contributing equally. It is the supervisor's responsibility to apply consequences

TABLE 6-7   Team Leader Behavior

Supervisory Behaviors	*Coaching Behaviors*
Hand out assignments	Develop a positive reinforcement plan
Tell people how to do a job	Give performance feedback
Keep people on task	Share information
Identify and punish poor performance	Mediate reinforcement between team members
Protect organizational information	Deliver positive reinforcement for decision-making, creative solutions, cooperation, and initiative

to team members in such a way that everybody is reinforced appropriately for his/her contributions to the team. It is critical that the criteria for receiving reinforcement and rewards are clear and achievable. If they are not, skepticism, cynicism, and bitterness among team members may result. The best way to empower team members is gradually and systematically.

You can encourage team development by providing support, promoting interaction, emphasizing goals, and facilitating task accomplishment. Be willing to share goal-setting, decision-making, problem-solving, and control with your group. Once you have an effective team, everyone's job will be easier, and more enjoyable—especially yours.

Most people want the chance to be a member of a winning team. They want to contribute to the group. You, as the supervisor, must facilitate and reinforce teamwork and provide your staff with the tasks and projects to challenge them successfully. You will also reap the benefits and satisfaction of team building and discover the value of teams. Teamwork is demanding of the individual members. Supervisors and team leaders need to be cognizant of this fact and appreciate the effort required.

Each team member must function within his or her scope of practice. Every state has a specific scope of practice for licensed nurses as well as for CNAs. These scopes are regulatory and identify what the practitioner can and cannot do. It is both illegal and unsafe to ask team members to do something outside their scopes of practice. It is also incumbent on every practitioner to be familiar with his or her professional scope of practice. Not knowing scope-of-practice requirements will not protect a nurse in a malpractice lawsuit. State scope-of-practice regulations are legal requirements of how nursing is practiced and/or what CNAs are allowed to do (or forbidden from doing).

Each person on the team has certain responsibilities to fulfill when working. Those responsibilities usually are determined by the charge nurse on each shift. Because each shift has different responsibilities depending on the time of day and the type of unit, these responsibilities vary between shifts. (See Table 6-8.) Each team member is responsible for tasks according to his or her individual scope of practice.

Characteristics of Effective Team Leaders

Effective team leaders:

- communicate.
- are open, honest, and fair.
- make decisions with input from others.
- act consistently.
- give team members the information they need to do their jobs.
- set goals and emphasize them.
- keep focused through follow-up.
- listen to feedback and ask questions.
- show loyalty to the company and to the team members.
- create an atmosphere for growth.
- have wide visibility.
- give praise and recognition.
- criticize constructively and address problems.
- develop plans.
- share mission and goals.
- display tolerance and flexibility.
- demonstrate assertiveness.
- exhibit willingness to change.
- treat team members with respect.
- make themselves available and accessible.
- want to take charge.
- accept ownership for team decisions.
- set guidelines for how team members are to treat one another.
- represent the team and fight the good fight when appropriate.

Adapted from *Supervisory Training Modules,* Beverly Health and Rehab., adapted 2005.

Characteristics of an Effective Team

- Team members share a sense of purpose or common goals, and each team member is willing to work toward achieving these goals.
- The team is aware of and interested in its own processes and in examining norms operating within the team.
- The team identifies its own resources and uses them, depending on its needs. The team willingly accepts the influence and leadership of members whose resources are relevant to the immediate task.
- Team members continually try to listen to and clarify what is being said and show interest in what others say and feel.
- Differences of opinion are encouraged and freely expressed. The team does not demand narrow conformity or adherence to formats that inhibit freedom of movement and expression.
- The team is willing to bring conflict to the surface and focus on it until it is resolved or managed in a way that does not reduce the effectiveness of those involved.
- The team exerts energy toward problem-solving rather than allowing its energy to be drained by interpersonal issues or competitive struggles.
- Roles are balanced and shared to facilitate both the accomplishment of tasks and feelings of team cohesion and morale.
- To encourage risk-taking and creativity, mistakes are treated as sources of learning rather than reasons for punishment.
- The team is responsive to the changing needs of its members and to the external environment to which it is related.
- Team members are committed to periodically evaluating the team's performance.
- Members identify with the team and consider it a source of both professional and personal growth.
- Developing a climate of trust is recognized as the crucial element for facilitating all of the above elements.

Adapted from *Supervisory Training Modules,* Beverly Health and Rehab., adapted 2005.

TABLE 6-8   Typical Patient-Care Responsibilities (scope varies by state)

Registered Nurse	LVN/LPN	CNA
Coordinate care of team	Provide meds or technical procedures as trained and directed by RN	Assist patients and provide activities of daily living as needed, ambulate and transport patients
Assess patients, determine interventions and evaluation	Report results of interventions to RN, collect data as directed, report changes in patient condition, reinforce education plan	Collect and report data and patient condition changes to RN
Create and administer patient education plan	Assist CNA with data collection and procedures	Assist LVN/LPN with procedures as needed

The team leader is charged with making appropriate decisions that result in effective use of the team. A successful team has all its members working together and communicating well with each other. Tasks are completed, not forgotten, and changing patient conditions are promptly reported and managed.

Additional members of a patient-care team include:

- Dietician
- Infection control nurse
- Pharmacist
- Physician
- Clinical case manager
- Discharge planner

Standards of practice and role-based competencies drive different roles, functions, and tasks. Standards of practice and competent performance are defined by several organizations, including hospitals as well as regulatory agencies. Standard practices and skill-based competencies are defined by hospital policy and directed toward the ongoing commitment to quality improvement and patient satisfaction.

Standards for performance are also defined by individual job descriptions for each team member. Facility job descriptions list specific tasks and functions for each role. Performance evaluations are geared to specific job description requirements, tasks, and functions for each role. Standards of practice are also defined by state and federal regulations. You can review the standards of competent performance for your state of licensure on your state board of nursing Web site.

Accountability is also a function of teamwork. Each team member is held accountable and must be responsible for carrying out physician orders within his or her scope of practice. Members of a team have accountability not only to the patient, but also to the patient's family, the physician, the organization, the payer, and other team members.

Commitment is part of being a team. Each team member must be committed to the goals of the team and the organization. Each team member is accountable for and committed to implementing the patient's plan of care within each discipline and scope of practice. Team members must use their skills to the overall benefit of the patient. A commitment also exists from each team member to the patient and the patient's family, as well as to providing a high quality of care. All members must be committed to positive patient outcomes as well as cost-effective patient care.

Newly constructed teams go through several stages before they work well together, some more quickly than others. In 1965, Bruce Tuckman created a model for team functioning that is well known in management circles (Marks, 1994). Tuckman lists four stages of team development:

- Forming: getting started, getting to know each other, not sure what to do.
- Storming: going in circles, having trouble working together, focused on end goal instead of process of getting work done.
- Norming: getting on course, now knowing each other, identifying goals, and working together.
- Performing: working full speed ahead, working together to achieve goals, using feedback to make changes, looking for ways to improve.

Even if you are a nurse manager and part of an administrative team, your team members still go through these four stages. Some teams are dysfunctional and never get out of the storming phase. Committees and unit teams that are effective have successfully worked through all four stages and remain in the performing stage for the long term. Whenever a new team member joins the group, it is common for the team to go back through storming and norming stages again before getting back to performing.

As with everything else related to nursing, communication is critical among team members. Staff and team members will perform functions that support the mission of the organization and unit if they:

- have clearly defined goals.
- recognize how they treat each other will affect how they relate to patients.
- recognize the team leader and his/her functions and responsibilities.
- agree on the purpose and functions of the team.
- are clear on who is responsible, who has authority, and who is accountable for what tasks and functions.
- have open and honest communication.
- deal with conflict honestly and openly.

- welcome and accept new members.
- value all team members.
- understand all team member roles and tasks and define them for the entire team.
- provide continual information within and for the team.

Teams work best if team leaders (usually the RN):

- support team members' sense of self-worth and the importance of each member's role.
- are open to ideas and suggestions for how to accomplish team workload.
- embrace high standards of performance that are clearly communicated.
- encourage all members to express ideas and value other members.
- ensure that team members have what they need to perform their role and tasks—equipment, knowledge, resources, and skills.
- coach team members at their particular level of ability to enhance performance (one-size coaching *does not* fit all).
- place emphasis on problem-solving, not blaming.
- recognize that obstacles and change are facts of life for teams.

It is important for team leaders and members to know when to:

- empower all team members.
- educate team members when conditions are new or changed.
- coach before, during, and after a first experience.
- counsel when problems damage performance.
- confront problems when they are persistent or when a person is failing.
- give feedback early and often.

Teams require personal communication, which is effective when:

- the goal is to create understanding.
- listening is more important than talking.
- nonverbal communication is 98% of process.
- two-way communication is preferred.
- one-way communication is used if necessary for a crisis.

Proper delegation to other team members occurs when:

- the team leader identifies the tasks to be delegated.
- team members know their responsibility is to complete tasks *and* report back to the team leader.

- it is within practice scope.
- unsavory tasks are not dumped.
- the team member is competent and has equipment/supplies to do the task.
- it is seen as an opportunity to teach team members new skills by demonstrating procedure or tasks.

For Your Toolkit

When working with a team, listening is more important than talking.

Effective Delegation

All supervisors and managers wonder at some point why they have so much work to complete and no one to assist them. Reasons for this perception include:

- I don't have enough time.
- I'd rather do it myself.
- I can't trust that a subordinate will do it correctly.
- I can't give my work to someone else because my boss will think I can't do it.
- It's my job.
- My subordinates already have too much to do.

No matter how effective you are as a supervisor, there is a limit to what you can accomplish yourself. Successful supervisors know when and what to delegate. Delegation is the assignment of authority for the completion of tasks to others. This allows completion and achievement of organizational goals. Effective supervisors learn the art of effective delegation, which results in win-win for both the supervisor and the subordinate.

One of the major concepts of delegation is to provide subordinates with the necessary information and authority to complete the tasks assigned, but you retain the responsibility for the final achievement of the goals or outcome. In doing this, you and your subordinates gain these benefits:

- Increased span of responsibility.
- Increased time to spend on planning.
- Staff development of subordinates.
- Increased motivation.
- Increased productivity and efficiency.

You win as a supervisor in that as you increase the responsibilities of your subordinates, you expand your own ability to manage more effectively through increased planning and decision-making. Your subordinates win through the application of skills they have learned and the empowerment gained in solving work problems. Both of you win when your value to the organization increases and the job satisfaction of the team is enhanced.

For Your Toolkit

> **As you increase the responsibilities of your subordinates, you expand your own ability to manage more effectively.**

Now that you understand the idea and value of delegation, how do you go about doing it? (See Table 6-9.) Many supervisors believe that delegating means assigning parts of their work they don't want to do to someone else. This is not delegating. It is dumping. To properly delegate to others you must first analyze what tasks you can safely, legally, and appropriately delegate. Consider training, certification, or licensure requirements when evaluating this. Determine the authority needed for the job and how much can be delegated. Consider such things as requesting information from others in the organization. Can your subordinate have access to the same information? Can s/he represent you?

You must then determine who the right person for the job is. Consider the following components.

- Does the work belong to a particular position?
- Does the task fit well with duties already performed, and thus would logically fit there? Who has the interest and/or ability?
- Who has the time?
- Is there a part-time person who could take on a new task and/or project?
- Is there a person whose workload has periods that are cyclic or lighter?
- How much control will be needed to ensure completion of the task delegated?
- Consider such things as establishing deadlines and check-in dates.

There are certain tasks as a supervisor you cannot delegate to others. These include things like discipline of subordinates or implementation of policies. Other examples are duties that require licensure or other specific credentialing or access to restricted data, such as payroll. You may not be able to delegate certain tasks to others because they have not been trained, such as completing a specific form or process. Tailor your delegation to fit your subordinates' abilities while allowing them the freedom to expand their skills.

You must also assess how much authority you can delegate to others based on the tasks assigned. For example, if you ask someone to investigate a work-related injury and make recommendations to prevent further incidents, then you must also ensure the person has the authority to conduct the investigation on your behalf. The nature and amount of authority delegated should be clearly defined and communicated to the subordinate. Delegating a portion of your authority to a subordinate does not relieve you of your responsibility to your boss and the organization to ensure the duties are properly completed.

In addition to determining what tasks you can delegate and how much delegated authority is needed to complete them, you must also establish controls for the type of work assigned. The methods you choose for control should be suited to the nature of the assignment and to the person to whom you have given the assignment. In some cases, periodic written reports may be required. In other cases, spot checks or verbal briefings may be enough. Once you have determined the controls needed to complete the tasks assigned, clearly communicate them to the subordinate.

Delegation has several steps to ensure delegation with effective results.

- Explain why the job is important.
- Explain the end results needed and let the staff member her/himself determine when the task will be completed.
- Delegate in terms of results and outcomes, not process or methods.
- Clearly define the authority and parameters delegated for completing the task.
- Agree on a deadline and time frame with the staff member.
- Ask for feedback to ensure the staff member understands the task completely.
- Provide for controls to ensure the staff member is on the right track.
- Follow up and check on progress yourself.
- Give support and an opportunity for the staff member to come back to you with questions.

Once an assignment is completed, be sure to give your subordinate credit for a job well done. You take responsibility if the assignment was less than successful. Let your subordinate know how well he or she did. If needed, review the original directions and discuss how to accomplish the assignment more effectively in the future. If the assignment was not completed accurately, find out what went wrong and why. Ask for your subordinate's feedback on the assignment, and ask if he or she would do another in the future.

The skills discussed will prepare you to be a more effective delegator. To prepare for your next opportunity to delegate, try imagining yourself preparing to delegate to

TABLE 6-9   Delegation Dos and Don'ts

Do	Don't
Encourage free flow of information to subordinates	Hoard information
Focus on results	Emphasize methods
Delegate through dialogue	Do all the talking yourself
Fix firm deadlines	Leave time frames unclear or uncertain
Make sure the person has all the necessary resources	Give assignments without the needed tools and information
Delegate the entire task to one person	Delegate half the task
Give advice without interfering	Fail to point out pitfalls
Build controls into the process of delegating	Impose controls as an afterthought
Back up the delegate in legitimate disputes	Leave delegates to fight their own battles on your behalf
Give the delegate full credit for his/her accomplishments	Hog the glory or look for a scapegoat

a specific subordinate. Picture the person, and think about the right approach to use in conveying an assignment to this person. Imagine how the person will respond. How will you go about getting feedback from this person on the assignment? How will you communicate the authority needed? What check dates and processes or deadlines will you establish? How will you ensure understanding of the assignment?

Evaluating and Critiquing Performance

Most people think of performance evaluations as something that happens once a year or if you make a mistake. Whereas supervisors and managers do formal performance evaluations, charge nurses and team leaders routinely evaluate performance of their team members. A performance evaluation is an opportunity to assess the demonstrated performance of team members and staff over a period of time. The evaluation communicates the assessment and expectations for the future. The document is a way to review the past and look toward the future using the performance evaluation process.

Numerous studies have been done in different industries about what is most important to people about working. Probably one of the best-known books on the subject is the *Art of Managing People* by Philip L. Hunsacker and Anthony L. Allesandria (1980). The two most frequently mentioned responses to all these studies were communication and recognition. People have a desire for accurate, timely information. People want to be in the loop. Not providing information makes staff members think you are deliberately keeping bad news from them. The second desire is to be

Turner Delegation Self-Assessment Checklist©

Check all that apply.

1. Your workload has prevented you from taking regular vacations.

2. You feel overworked frequently.

3. You leave jobs unfinished.

4. You take work home most nights and weekends.

5. You always seem to have more work than your subordinates.

6. Planning is a low-priority task for you.

7. You have no time for outside activities.

8. In the past week, you have engaged in detail work that isn't in your job.

9. You frequently do your subordinates' work for them.

10. Crises and problems are more common in your job than opportunities.

11. Often you haven't had time to explain fully a task to a subordinate.

12. You frequently have problems meeting your boss's deadlines.

13. You like to keep your hand in your old job.

14. You are a perfectionist—and proud of it!

(continues)

Turner Delegation Self-Assessment Checklist© (continued)

15. You wish you had more time in your personal life.

16. You can't think of your top three current work goals.

17. You believe in giving subordinates only the information they need to do their specific jobs.

18. You rarely elicit the opinions of your subordinates about anything.

19. In your opinion, your subordinates are not to be trusted with too much information.

20. It is hard for you to accept ideas offered by someone else.

21. You get the feeling that sometimes your subordinates are trying to undermine you.

22. You believe your subordinates are coasting.

23. Your subordinates think how something is done is more important than what is achieved.

24. Your staff refuses to make any decisions without consulting you first.

25. Your staff comes to you for advice on their work more than necessary.

26. Your staff exceeds their authority regularly.

27. Your staff acts according to the literal rather than the spirit of an assignment.

Turner Delegation Self-Assessment Checklist© (continued)

28. Sometimes, your staff consults with you after the fact about significant actions.

29. None of your staff could fill in for you if you got run over by a bus.

30. Your staff turns work assignments back to you and you accept them.

31. Your staff wouldn't work at all if you weren't there to push them to do tasks.

32. Your staff has skills essentially unchanged from a year ago.

33. Staff rarely comes to you with new ideas or new ways of doing their jobs.

Adapted from Beverly Health and Rehab. Turner Healthcare Associates, Inc., © 1999.

recognized for a job well done. A pat on the back is a way of formally recognizing employees and makes them aware that the supervisor knows they did a good job. Staff expects communication and recognition from their direct supervisor. Even if you are not a designated supervisor, but function in the role of team leader or charge nurse, staff will expect informal feedback about their performance.

The reason actual performance evaluation is such a significant process is that it addresses the important employee needs for communication and recognition. It gives a supervisor the chance to communicate accurately how a staff member is performing. It is also a time for both the staff member and the supervisor to restate expectations and set new goals. Performance evaluations give the supervisor an opportunity to recognize staff performance and praise strengths as well as identify areas to improve. This should be happening on an ongoing basis so that getting a performance evaluation should have no surprises for the staff member.

Communication is a large part of the performance evaluation process. As discussed in the section on effective communication, words are important, but how we communicate beyond words makes up the bulk of our communication. To be accurate in communication in the performance evaluation process means that the supervisor or team leader must accurately assess the staff member's performance. This means concentrating on job performance—not on the staff member's personality—when making the assessment.

For Your Toolkit

> **Getting a performance evaluation should mean no surprises for the staff member.**

A performance evaluation can be thought of as a triangle. (See Figure 6-1.) It must be accurate, communicated, and timely. Most employees know when their performance evaluations are due because they are important to them. Completing them in a timely fashion builds credibility for the supervisor and the respect of employees. When communicating to staff, be sure that the communication is not one-sided. It is an exchange between you and your associate. In this process the supervisor should solicit input, comments, and suggestions from the employee.

When completing a performance evaluation, start the process early. Be on time with a complete evaluation. Review the employee's file for commendations, discipline, and memos for follow-up. Do this so you can consider the total performance. Remember that it is a positive thing if a staff member overcomes a previous performance problem. Review the employee's job description to ensure it is still accurate and to assist you in considering the entire job and all its various responsibilities. Assess job performance objectively, not the staff member's personality or attitude. Assess how the employee has performed the job, not just whether you think he or she is a nice person.

Your objectivity is enhanced when there are job duties that can be counted or measured, for example, attendance or number of students preceptored. Consider the staff member's performance for the entire time period. Do not base your assessment on only the most recent weeks or months. You are assessing performance for the entire year. Use specific examples to describe positive and negative performance. Use examples to clarify and support your position and promote credibility.

Schedule the time to meet with the employee. This demonstrates your respect for the process and the staff member. This also gives the staff member time to prepare for the meeting. Review the job description in advance. Consider all aspects of the job. Meet in a private and in a comfortable place behind closed doors. This eliminates interruptions and maintains privacy. Explain the purpose of the discussion and set the stage for an open, honest, cordial discussion. Praise the employee's strengths and identify areas to improve. Balance the discussion with comments on both areas.

Encourage the staff member to participate with input and comments. The contact should not be a one-sided monologue. The discussion requires input from the staff member as well as the supervisor. Give the employee every opportunity to partic-

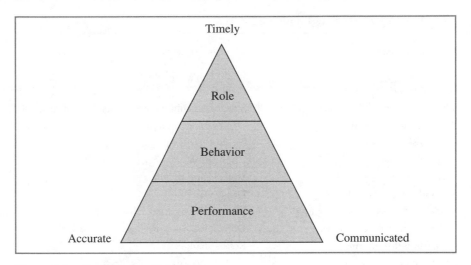

Figure 6-1   Performance Evaluation

ipate in the process by your listening and not interrupting. Focus your comments on the employee's performance, not personality. There should be no surprises for the employee during this discussion. Recognition and corrective action should have taken place as soon as needed—not be saved for the performance evaluation meeting.

Avoid confrontation and argument with the employee. Listen with objectivity, and stress performance, not personality or attitude. Assess the employee's past demonstrated performance, but emphasize the future and professional growth. Restate your expectations. Don't save communicating expectations for these meetings, but rather use the time to reinforce those you have already shared with the employee. Set new goals, considering progress, growth, future, and employee development. Establish a plan and timetable to meet those objectives with the employee. Be specific, and monitor that the timetable is being met by the employee. Be sure the employee is aware of the effects of not satisfying performance standards. Employees deserve to know the consequences of not performing up to expectations. Remember to say "thank you" for your associate's participation in the meeting and his or her contribution for the year.

There are specific ways to describe both positive and negative employee behaviors in a written performance evaluation. Be sure always to support the adjectives used with specific examples of the staff member's behavior. Table 6-10 lists some words and phrases that can be used for describing both positive and negative behaviors.

Providing Discipline to Staff Members

Formal, progressive discipline is a last resort for sharing expectations with employees. If employee performance is a problem, numerous discussions and clarification of

TABLE 6-10   Describing Employee Behavior

Positive Behavior	*Negative Behavior*
Methodical	Needs many explanations
Generates enthusiasm	Perfectionist
Willing to accept difficult assignments	Slow to get things done; resists difficult materials
Pays attention to deadlines	Overreacts to criticism
Avoids risks	Tends to daydream
Gets tasks done	Unprepared
Accountable for own work	Shifts blame to others
Sets and completes goals	Disorganized
Sensitive when showing disapproval	Unfriendly to patients; inefficient
Willing to help others succeed	Does not check work before submission
Obtains needed information	Resists changes
Shares information with others	Disrupts meetings
Maintains high standards	Takes shortcuts
Flexible	Sensitive to criticism
Becomes adaptable to those in authority	Resists participation in team; displays superior attitude
Gives recognition to others	Overuses enthusiasm
Takes on challenges	Displays frustration
Works calmly in unpredictable environment	Becomes soft and persuadable under pressure
Good organizer	Easily intimidated
Good listener; team player	Fails to communicate information, directions, feelings
Innovative	Shows little imagination
Makes good decisions quickly	Makes decisions too fast
Diplomatic with people	Abrupt with others

performance expectations should take place before the disciplinary process begins. Just the word "discipline" strikes fear in even the most confident managers. It doesn't need to. Although you probably will never look forward to taking disciplinary action, you can get to a point where you are comfortable and confident in what you are doing.

Progressive discipline is used to correct a deficiency in conduct, performance, or a violation of policy in an effort to get someone to meet established standards of job performance in order to preserve his or her employment and to encourage that person to behave sensibly and safely at work. Progressive discipline is actually a continually forward-focused instruction and education process. In using discipline as a form of training, it would be appropriate to reward with praise and advancement staff who observe facility rules and who meet or exceed job performance standards. It is also appropriate to discipline staff members who do not follow facility rules and meet performance standards, so that they can be educated on acceptable performance and behavior. Staff needs to hear that what they are doing is right, as well as receive feedback on problematic personnel issues.

Chaos would ensue if there were no rules in the workplace. Most staff see discipline as a way to preserve order and safety. It is reasonable and expectable that an organization have staff working toward common organizational goals and standards. Staff expects just and equal treatment, in which discipline is in line with a performance problem or misconduct. The action must fit the infraction, and all staff members who are disciplined for an action must be treated equitably and fairly. Staff expects reasonable policies and consistent application of those policies.

Most staff members are conscientious, dependable, and want to do a good job. They infrequently or never require disciplinary action. When an individual has a performance problem, it is generally an isolated incident and is quickly corrected with counseling or disciplinary action. A small percentage of staff causes most disciplinary problems. Ongoing performance and behavior problems can result from lack of interest, lack of effort, problems getting along with others, or problems at home. Part of a supervisor's job is to help staff adjust to their work. If the supervisor is a good leader, shows a sincere interest in staff, and makes work enjoyable, the staff is far less likely to break rules or cause problems. Each facility has specific progressive discipline policies. If you are a supervisor and are expected to administer progressive discipline, become familiar with the policy *before* you need to implement it. During the stress and urgency of an actual disciplinary situation is not when you want to be reading the policy for the first time.

Most facilities have a policy that starts with a clarification of performance expectations. If problems continue, the employee receives a verbal warning. Facilities use either one or two written warnings before an employee is terminated. There are instances where termination is immediate for gross misconduct, such as threatening another employee, being under the influence of a chemical substance, or lying during the hiring interview or on the employment application.

One of the most important aspects of the disciplinary process is to determine whether it is truly justified. A complete and impartial investigation into the situation must be conducted before discipline is applied. Usually, the more information at your disposal, the clearer the decision generally is. Once your investigation has revealed that an employee has committed a known policy violation, it is time to ascertain what action to take. Employees are often placed on suspension until the investigation is completed. The usual time frame for this type of suspension is up to three regularly scheduled days, but this varies by facility.

Verbal warnings are not mandatory but are usually issued prior to a written warning, particularly if the infraction is minor in nature. Written warnings are usually issued once the employee has received a verbal warning already and failed to correct the deficiency, has committed a more serious infraction which warrants more than a verbal warning, or has one or more prior verbal or written warnings. Termination happens infrequently and is used when no other alternative exists to deal with the infraction. Termination is rarely immediate and is usually contemplated only after an investigation is completed.

If you must conduct a disciplinary meeting with an employee, schedule it after the investigation is complete. Make an appointment and ensure complete privacy. Complete the necessary paperwork prior to the meeting and have it ready, including paychecks and forms if it is a termination. Review the paperwork with the employee and explain why the action is being taken. Get the necessary signatures and provide the employee with a copy of the disciplinary action document. If the employee has been terminated, have him or her discreetly escorted out of the facility. After the meeting has taken place, document the conversation, and submit all paperwork for additional signatures and processing.

Progressive discipline is not much fun for anyone involved in it. It is much easier to coach and supervise employees instead of disciplining them. Remember that proper training, education, and supervisory support will go a long way in preventing the need for disciplinary action. Discipline should be used only as necessary and then as a corrective action. It is much easier to stop a small problem and avoid much larger issues.

Decision-Making

Part of being a successful manager or supervisor is to have the competencies needed to achieve goals. Robert Katz identified three essential management skill sets: technical, human, and conceptual (Robbins, 1996). Technical skills are those that encompass the ability to apply specialized knowledge or expertise. Extensive formal education is needed. Human skills are those that demonstrate ability to work with, understand, and motivate other people, both individually and in groups. Many managers are technically proficient but interpersonally incompetent. Because managers get things done through other people, they must have good human skills in order to communicate, motivate, and delegate effectively. Managers who are poor listeners, who are unable to understand the needs of others, or who have difficulty managing conflicts will not be effective managers.

A key concept that affects managers' abilities to get things done is their ability to manage problem-solving and make decisions. Problem-solving and decision-making are based on perception, defined as the process by which individuals organize and interpret their sensory impressions in order to give meaning to their environment. However, what someone perceives as reality can be substantially different from what is real (Robbins, 1996).

There are numerous factors that influence perception. Attitudes, motives, interests, experience, and expectations all affect how people view a situation. In a given situation, issues like time and setting (personal or workplace) influence perception. Novelty, motion, sounds, size, background, and proximity all influence individual perceptions about a given experience. These factors become significant when managers are evaluating workplace situations and making decisions.

For Your Toolkit

People don't *see* reality. They *interpret* what they see and call it reality.

There is a link between perception and decision-making. Decision-making occurs as a reaction to a problem. A discrepancy exists between a current state of affairs and a desired state, requiring consideration of alternative courses of action. Unfortunately, most problems don't come neatly packaged with a label on them. One person's problem is another person's satisfactory state of affairs. Every decision requires interpretation and evaluation of information. Data must be screened, processed, and interpreted to allow evaluation.

Because people perceive experiences differently, no two people approach decision-making the same way. However, there is an optimal way of making decisions. The Optimizing Decision Making Model (Robbins, 1996) describes how individuals should behave in order to maximize an outcome. There are six steps to this process.

The first step requires recognition that a decision needs to be made. The existence of a problem brings about this recognition.

The second step is to identify the decision criteria. In this step, the only criteria evaluated are those the decision-maker considers relevant. Therefore, different people will have different decision criteria. In health care, important criteria are length of stay, productivity, overtime, staffing matrices, and patient outcomes.

The third step is to allocate weights to the criteria. Not all criteria are equally important. It is necessary to weight the factors in order to prioritize their importance in the decision. The decision-maker can weight criteria numerically or with other measures. The result allows decision-makers to prioritize the relevant criteria and to indicate the criteria's relative degree of importance.

The fourth step is to develop alternatives. The decision-maker lists all the alternatives that could possibly succeed in resolving the problem. No attempt is made to appraise alternatives, but only to list them.

Step five involves evaluating alternatives. Once the alternatives have been identified, the decision-maker must evaluate each one. The strengths and weaknesses of each alternative

Steps in Optimizing Decision-Making

1. Ascertain the need for a decision.
2. Identify the decision criteria.
3. Allocate weights to the criteria.
4. Develop alternatives.
5. Evaluate alternatives.
6. Select the best alternative.

will become evident when compared against the criteria and weights established in the previous steps. Evaluation of each alternative is done by appraising it against the weighted criteria.

The sixth and last step is to select the best alternative. Technically, this should be easy. The decision-maker simply chooses the alternative that generated the highest total score. However, good decisions in the healthcare industry are rarely so clearly identified. For most people, the optimizing model is usually the exception, not the rule. Few important decisions are simple or unambiguous. Some managers look for solutions that suffice rather than optimize, which injects biases and prejudices into the decision process. Others rely on intuition. Most managers and supervisors attempt to make rational decisions.

Rationality refers to choices that are consistent and value maximizing. Rational decision-making implies that the decision-maker can be fully objective and logical, with a clear goal. Rationality and the optimizing model assume that there is no conflict over goals and that all options are known and identified, with constant and unchanging criteria and preferences. Rational decision-makers would choose the alternative that gives the maximum benefits or maximizes the decision outcome. But decision-making is not just an analysis of facts. There is an element of gut feel to the process, especially when it comes to knowing when you have reached the point where you have sufficient facts on which to base a decision with a minimum of risk. This gut feel often separates the effective from the ineffective manager (Robbins, 1996).

Problem-Solving

Problem-solving requires good decision-making. The end result of decision-making by individuals and groups is driven by their ability to solve problems. Although we would like to think otherwise, problems exist for all groups that work together. Robbins (1996) identifies a nine-step process of problem-solving.

The first step is to identify the apparent problem versus the root problem. The apparent problem is what you think caused the issue. The root problem is what actually went wrong. The root problem is rarely the apparent problem. It is important to uncover the root problem, because it may be much more significant than the apparent problem. Robbins calls this the "iceberg effect." Identifying the root cause of a problem allows all factors to be evaluated and corrected and minimizes placing blame on specific individuals.

The second step is to identify the key players needed in the resolution of the problem. Problem-solving teams try to bring all involved or affected parties together. The group then can define the problem in a statement, which is the third step. This statement is not always the same as the apparent problem.

For Your Toolkit

The apparent problem is what you think caused the issue. The root problem is what actually went wrong.

The fourth step is to collect and analyze data about the situation in order to resolve the issue. There are organizations that continually collect data but rarely do anything with it. This is known as "analysis paralysis" and does not move toward problem-solving and resolution.

The fifth step is to share the data with *all* the stakeholders. This means sharing the data (not *just* the interpretation of the data) with *everyone* potentially affected by the problem and resolution. This is usually a lot of people. Those who schedule meetings tend to limit the number of participants and focus only on having managers attend. Unfortunately, it is the front-line staff that usually has firsthand experience with the problem and can help with potential solutions. Be sure to include everyone who can help resolve a problem.

The sixth step occurs once the larger group is gathered. Explain both the apparent problem and the root cause, if known, and have all participants brainstorm solutions. During brainstorming, include all suggestions, no matter how outlandish. Brainstorming is the time for listing all ideas without judgment or commentary. The group can evaluate them later.

The seventh step is the elimination technique, which involves isolating the best ideas. The eighth step involves creating a plan of action. Inform *all* stakeholders of this plan and ask for feedback *before* implementing it. Make revisions to the plan and then determine an implementation strategy that works for *all* the stakeholders, which is the ninth step. Faulty implementation of a plan can make a good decision ineffective.

Effective implementation of a plan can make a debatable choice successful. Solving the root problem is only half of the solution. Implementation of a plan is what will complete the cycle.

When teams work together on problem-solving, they often get stuck in terms of their ability to move through a problem to the solution. You can identify the team behaving as stuck by the symptoms listed here.

- Lack of progress
- Canceling meetings
- Angry exchanges between members
- Loss of energy
- Helplessness/victimization
- Lack of purpose/identity
- Dishonesty and lack of candor
- Cynicism and mistrust
- Personal attacks made behind team members' backs
- Finger pointing

Getting the team unstuck involves revisiting the purpose of the team and identifying small wins and progress steps. Sometimes you can also search out new information and approaches. In rare situations, you may need to consider changing team members, including the team leader.

Many times getting stuck is caused by conflict. This is usually because team members have different ideas of what the team goal is or how to get there. Because tasks moving toward problem resolution affect more than one person/group, what works successfully in one part of the organization is a disaster in another. Team members can get frustrated if their unit does not obtain scarce resources. Hospital organizational structure may also impede solutions and problem-solving due to dysfunctional senior management teams or bureaucratic delays. All of these issues can cause conflict for teams.

When managing the conflict in a team, remember that problem-solving efforts must include members from conflicting groups. This does not mean that groups should point fingers at each other, but rather calmly discuss their perceptions and differences. It is also helpful to rotate team members among different teams to facilitate understanding. The best example I experienced in my career was an RN working in the intensive care unit (ICU) who transferred to the Emergency Department (ED) as a floating or *per diem* staff member. Once an ICU nurse understands how the ED works, s/he will never again argue with an ED calling the ICU to admit a patient immediately because of others coming in the door. The most helpful strategy for conflict resolution I have used involves refocusing team members on shared group goal(s). Ask what's best for the patient, and that will usually get discussion flowing in the right direction again. Team members tend not to argue when the focus is on patient outcomes.

It is important to remind team members of their commitment to the group during a conflict-management stage. Take some time to define each team member's responsibility to meeting stated goals of the unit or group. Define the expected outcomes and time frame for achieving them. Be sure to revisit conflict resolution if a team member is not willing or not able to meet team responsibilities. Have the team revisit the goals and expected outcomes of care on a regular basis to ensure that the quality-improvement process is inherent in daily practice.

For Your Toolkit

Keep the focus on patient outcomes.

Team conflict can also be triggered by transition and change. Change makes many people uncomfortable. Change involves letting go of old practices and expectations but can also mean doing your job more effectively. Change often causes fear, grief, and loss. Some people adapt better to change than others. People are like popcorn, and pop (adapt) to change and new ideas at different times.

Because bedside-care management is mandatory in today's healthcare environment, a team approach is necessary for that to occur. Care management is critical to achieve positive patient outcomes and a perfect fit for the patient and for a team approach. Bedside-care management enhances physician, payer, patient, and clinician satisfaction. It is a different concept from focusing team-member efforts on daily tasks. Team members must remember to incorporate tasks within an entire perspective on patient-care planning. Keep the perspective on the total patient, not just on tasks. Tasks are not all that registered nurses do, although performance of tasks within the scope of practice is inherent in job responsibilities each day. Bedside-care management improves the use of resources, increases job satisfaction, and decreases patient length of stay. A team approach means true care management for the patient.

Chapter 7

Encouraging Others to Succeed

"An expert was once a beginner"

—DR. PATRICIA BENNER

Effective Mentoring

All professional nurses need special insight, understanding, wisdom, and information that a mentor or executive coach can provide. Coaches and mentors can help individual nurses successfully navigate multiple challenges, changes, and demands. The need for coaching and mentoring has never been more apparent for leaders at all levels because how people progress within their careers is changing (Gates & Rubano, 2004).

Webster's 9th edition defines *mentoring* as a trusted counselor or guide, tutor or coach, preceptor or teacher. According to Hein and Nicholson, "Mentoring occurs when a senior person (the mentor), in terms of age and/or experience, undertakes to provide information, advice and emotional support for a junior person in a relationship lasting over an extended period of time and marked by substantial emotional commitment by both parties" (Gates & Rubano, 2004).

Examples of mentoring in nursing include student nurses by experienced RNs, a new manager by an experienced manager, or orientation of a new employee by a

Characteristics of Mentoring

- Coaching
- Teaching
- Listening
- Providing advice
- Providing situational evaluation
- Making suggestions
- Role-playing
- Sponsoring
- Protecting
- Supporting
- Encouraging
- Affirming
- Inspiring
- Challenging
- Counseling
- Clarifying
- Accepting
- Communicating and interrelating
- Being kind
- Being patient
- Offering praise and constructive criticism
- Providing a mirror for views of self

buddy. There is a difference between mentoring and precepting. Precepting is a formal role, covered in a separate section.

Mentoring is not power-driven, authoritarian "my way or no way," or punitive. Mentoring is not something you are mandated to do in your career—forced compliance is not required. Mentoring is something you choose to do, and you accept the mentee completely, without judgment of his or her choices or behaviors.

Nurses interested in mentoring usually like sharing what they know. They are willing to teach, and enjoy working with students, new grads, and new employees. They accept the time commitment to work with mentees. Successful mentors are able to evaluate outcomes and to be kind, fair, empathetic, and objective. They are willing to share their own good and bad experiences because "Good judgment comes from experience. Experience comes from bad judgment." Mentors can assess how mentees best learn and provide praise and supportive criticism. Mentors are willing to influence others and to stretch and push mentees to grow and learn. They help mentees develop a realistic picture of themselves and their skills.

There is an interface between mentoring, professionalism, and career development. Professionalism includes accountability, responsibility, training, knowledge, role-modeling, critical-thinking, collegiality, being a team player, and the ability to influence others. Mentors can assist other nurses in their professional development. Mentoring is part of being a good leader. It is the function of a leader to be a role model, to teach, and to share what he/she knows with those who follow behind. Mentees are the future of nursing, and it is up to us to help them create their own personal path.

For Your Toolkit

Mentoring is part of being a good leader.

To navigate challenges in the workplace, as well as to do successful career planning, most people find benefits in using a coach or mentor. The old metaphor of climbing the corporate ladder is being replaced by a metaphor of moving out and around different branches of a large tree. Many mid-level managers and nurse executives are looking at nontraditional paths by which to pursue their career development. These moves can be a lateral move followed by an upward move, then another lateral move.

There is a difference between coaching and mentoring. Mentoring involves a personal relationship outside the supervisor–employee relationship. It may last for long periods of time or across the span of a career. Mentoring is career-focused and relates to professional development outside a mentee's current span of skills. Mentors provide both personal and professional support. Mentor relationships often cross job boundaries. Mentoring is focused on developing one's career and learning through someone else's expertise. Mentoring relationships include large areas of career development and require a long commitment over time. Mentoring usually creates relationships of value personally and professionally to both the mentee and mentor (Gates & Rubano, 2004).

Mentors can be active and passive. Active mentors are those who are willing to coach you as you progress. Passive mentors are role models you can emulate. You need both types in nursing. (See Chapter 3 on career development.)

Mentoring comes with responsibilities on you as a mentor. There is a commitment to the mentee of time and sharing. You must be caring, knowledgeable, and willing to share your own experiences. You need patience and the ability to validate others, while not taking their rejection of your suggestions personally. Although many mentors are in leadership positions, it is not necessary to be a manager in order to be an effective mentor. One of my mentors throughout my career has been a diploma-program staff nurse.

When you mentor others, you discuss situations and potential challenges. Your role is to listen and advise the mentee. You may write responses for specific requests for information or review certain materials. You meet and network with the mentee, providing sponsorship, introductions, and opportunities. Being a mentor allows you to share your knowledge, influence others, role-model professional behavior, assist with career development, and make a difference by helping someone change his/her life.

Effective Coaching

Although coaching may play a part in mentoring, executive coaching is usually more formal. Coaching is a process by which the coach works with an individual nurse to identify or suggest ways of changing performance to improve results. Coaching usually is focused on developing individuals within their current job or position. The coach and the nurse requesting the coaching usually have a specific agenda or skills to review. The coach assesses the nurse's individual skills and performance and helps develop an action plan that will allow the individual to achieve those goals. This is a very structured process and involves advanced, complex skills to help the individual nurse expand his/her capacity and take more effective actions. Coaching is usually a short-term commitment and may revolve around specific job skills the nurse wishes to improve (Gates & Rubano, 2004).

Every nurse is able to coach nurses who aspire to higher levels of competency and performance. It is part of the professional nursing role to assist others along the learning continuum to increase knowledge and skills. Mentoring nurses is a gift that each of us offers other nurses, using experience and wisdom to fully develop talents in the leaders that will follow us.

Effective Precepting*

Precepting means showing someone else how to perform your role. A preceptor is selected on the basis of the individual's work skills, knowledge of the unit/department, aptitude for teaching, and willingness to participate in orienting new employees. It is helpful to train preceptors before they begin.

A preceptor is a competent, proficient, or expert registered nurse with a special area of expertise, who is assigned or volunteers to help a novice or advanced beginner-level nursing student (Benner, Tanner, & Chesla, 1996). The preceptor guides and facilitates the student through the learning activities required to achieve the clinical course objectives. The preceptor actively participates in the evaluation of a student's clinical performance, though the final judgment always rests with the clinical educator for the course.

An effective preceptor demonstrates a high level of knowledge, clinical proficiency, and professionalism, and serves as a clinical instructor for new employees and students in the clinical setting. A preceptor also assists with the transition to the clinical environment in order to ensure quality patient services and maintains organizational standards and continuity of patient care in a cost-effective manner.

---

*The author wishes to thank Heather McCarthy, RN, MS, CNOR, Director of Surgical Services, Enloe Medical Center, Chico, California, for her contributions to this section.

For Your Toolkit

Precepting means showing someone else how to perform your role. It is a key retention strategy.

A preceptor's responsibilities include role model, facilitator, educator, and evaluator. Preceptors may provide input to unit-based orientation content and design. They are also encouraged to give input to general nursing orientation design and delivery. Preceptors evaluate the new orientee's performance and participate in planning activities when skill development is indicated. The preceptor assesses competencies only for topics in which s/he has documented competency. Preceptors provide the orientee with feedback and document the orientee's competencies by using competency checklists.

The educational level and clinical expertise of the preceptor should be greater than that of the student. Therefore, the education preparation for preceptors of baccalaureate students should be a BSN or higher degree. The minimal clinical experience expected is two years of full-time employment in the special clinical area. This does not have to be two years with a specific organization. In California, the preceptor must have a clear, current, active RN license. The department's nurse director/manager and clinical educator must agree to the employee serving as a preceptor.

A preceptor can be selected by the department manager, clinical educator, student, self, nursing school faculty member, or another preceptor. Nominations should be in writing or on the appropriate form for your facility. Preceptor nominations can also be made by verbal communication, such as by telephone or by written communication, such as e-mail, fax, letter, or note.

The preceptor is a resource person, facilitator, clinical role model, educator, and consultant to the student. The primary role is to provide a learning environment where the student can meet course and individual learning objectives. Preceptors have specific responsibilities, which differ from those of the unit manager or supervisor. Preceptors can work with student nurses and also with new employees.

In most situations the student/orientee will need to match the preceptor schedule rather than the other way around. In rare situations, the preceptor may designate another unit staff member to assist the student. The designee must be an RN with sufficient experience to assist the student. The preceptor (or designee) is continuously available when the student is in the clinical setting.

The responsibilities of the preceptor are to:

- assist the student/orientee by arranging opportunities and resources to obtain learning experiences appropriate to the course and individual learning objectives.

- assist the student in developing learning objectives. This includes advising the student of possible learning opportunities.
- sign the student's individual learning objectives following negotiation for appropriate learning experiences.
- assist students/orientees in orientation to the facility. This includes philosophy, policies, procedures, and expectations of the agency. Examples include dress code, special equipment, emergency situations (fire, disaster, and codes), documentation, charting, medication administration and documentation, access to the computer system for nursing documentation and retrieval of information, and telephone and fax use.
- verify student attendance.
- provide ongoing evaluation of student performance to the student and to the clinical educator.
- meet with the student midterm and end of term to discuss and document student achievement or lack of achievement of course and individual learning objectives. This is documented on the student learning contract.
- notify the student and faculty member at any time during the course that a course or individual learning objective is not met, or when a student has not made sufficient progress toward reaching an objective.
- evaluate the student's learning in conjunction with the clinical educator, based on course and individual learning objectives.
- evaluate the preceptor's own experience of the nursing course.

The role of the preceptor is crucial to the success of the new employee or student nurse. The nursing organization culture must value and support the role by providing a formal structure for the process. Because nursing students are potential facility employees, every effort should be made to make them feel confident and welcome and to ensure competency. An effective preceptor program using trained experienced preceptors will result in increased nurse retention in healthcare facilities.

Chapter 8
Workplace Transition

Entering the Nursing Workforce After Taking Time Off

It is common for nurses to take time off to have children or care for an elderly parent and then return to the workforce when their children are older or the parent has passed away. After a few years outside the workforce, it is natural to feel awkward about getting back into the work environment. Even if you were extremely accomplished and competent, you may feel a bit shaky about your skills and out of touch with the nursing profession.

Relax and have faith in your abilities. Remember, you had what it takes and that hasn't changed. If you look, sound, and act confident and professional, most employers will believe you are hirable. Don't apologize for taking the time off. If you traveled around the world or did research, you wouldn't apologize, so don't apologize for having a baby or taking care of a parent. Expect that employers will ask tough questions about your job gaps. Look at the questions as a chance to prove your mettle.

Don't second-guess your skills or credibility. Just try to update your knowledge and find a way to practice your skills. Some nursing schools will let alumni come in and use the skills lab to practice skills like IVs, Foleys, and nasogastric tubes. Get online and read the latest nursing journals and do some industry research. Find out what the latest regulations and the hottest healthcare issues are.

Call folks you know who are still working in health care. Ask them about the latest products and issues. Reconnect with co-workers and see what they can tell you about patient care issues and what jobs are open. Tell them you are going back to work and to let you know if they hear of a job opportunity for which you might qualify.

When you interview for jobs, ask about being assigned to a preceptor for assistance with getting your skills up to speed. Competency checklists are mandated in most facilities, so you can document what skills you are going to need some assistance with refreshing, and what you can do well. Nursing tasks are a bit like bike riding . . . they come back as soon as you start pedaling.

Keep in mind that specialty nursing skills are always in demand, and never more so than in a shortage. You can make a strong, positive impression on potential employers before they even see your resume. This means networking and making personal connections first. You can always meet potential employers by attending job or career fairs for nurses or attending specialty conferences. You can talk during breaks or lunch at a conference with those employers who would be too busy at work.

For Your Toolkit

Nursing tasks are a bit like bike riding . . . they come back as soon as you start pedaling.

Ask everyone you meet about job opportunities, and make sure all the people you talk with know you are interested in rejoining the workforce. Talking to strangers is a *good* idea when it comes to career development. Bring business cards with your contact information, and remember to write a thank-you note if someone provides you with a lead or other assistance.

For Your Toolkit

Talking to strangers is a *good* idea when it comes to career development.

No matter what kind of job you are looking for, you will need to have basic computer literacy. If you do not have computer skills, sign up for a class at your local community college or adult education center. This will be an important skill set to identify or discuss when you schedule a formal interview.

You may also want to schedule an informational interview. Informational interviews give you a chance to interview a nurse in a role in which you are interested. You will be able to find out how much additional education or specialty training is required, as well as get an unbiased view about the benefits and drawbacks of the position. You may also be able to arrange to job shadow that person for a day, so you can really see what the role would be like if you were in it.

You may not want to ask directly for a job during these informational interviews. But if you have made a positive and strong impression, chances are s/he will tell you about potential job opportunities. Be sure to follow up these interviews with a thank-you note and a copy of your updated resume.

When you are re-entering the workforce after time off, you may want to seek professional advice on setting up your resume to best highlight your past experience and skills. Keep in mind that the best facilities to approach if you are re-entering the workforce may be small organizations with flexible hiring policies, woman-owned businesses, and facilities with a "family friendly" reputation.

You may also wish to enroll in a nursing refresher/reentry program offered by some nursing schools. If you select this option, be sure the curriculum meets the criteria of the state board of nursing where the course is offered.

When You Get Sidelined in Your Career

Do you feel out of the loop at work and seem to be watching work going on around you? If you are informed of decisions only after the fact, or find out about meetings you should be invited to and weren't, you could be getting sidelined. According to Marilyn Moats Kennedy (1996), employees can be sidelined and pushed out of the mainstream without being aware of it. Organizations will tolerate an employee out of the mainstream only for a short period of time before the employee is terminated or laid off. Consider some of these questions listed by Kennedy:

- Has anything happened on the job in the past week that surprised you?
- Do people stop talking when you approach?
- Are your decisions overruled by your peers?
- Does your boss send you messages through your subordinates?
- Are you rarely asked for your opinion or input?
- Are your telephone calls rarely returned?
- Do people request your voicemail rather than trying to reach you directly?

If you answered "yes" to any of these questions, your job may be at risk. If you have pulled back at work because you are frustrated or exhausted, it may be visible to those near you.

The realization that you are on the outside comes so gradually it may be almost imperceptible until one event makes it plain to all. At that point, it is usually too late. Hanging back, withdrawing from the craziness, or just hiding out in your workspace should be warning signs that you are approaching burnout, or that your problems are visible to others, according to Kennedy.

You need to take action quickly. Talk to your boss and buy some time. Volunteer for a new project. Reconnect with co-workers. Most important of all—don't kid yourself about what is happening. The longer inaction is observed, the fewer the choices. Don't put yourself in the position of having your job eliminated due to lack of productivity or inability to work with others.

Layoffs/Reduction in Force

The scenarios for layoffs are always tough. They usually go something like this: your nurse manager calls you to her office. She seems uneasy, doesn't make much small talk, and eventually gets around to telling you your position has been eliminated. No matter how it is presented, being laid off always comes as a personal blow. As a veteran of four layoffs myself, I know just how bad it feels. Although no one can make it go away, you can at least get what you deserve. By remembering the following tips, you can ensure that you get maximum severance pay and benefits, as well as favorable references from your current employer (Turner, 1995a).

Take a deep breath and prepare to be successful at being out of a job. Don't take the layoff personally. Many excellent long-term employees have been laid off as the healthcare economic climate changes. As much as you feel like it, don't lash out. Getting angry at your manager, human resources representatives, or administrator may reduce your negotiating power. Don't try to get even because you never know when you will have to work with that person again. Everybody knows everyone in nursing. Don't burn any bridges; you may need them later.

Pack up all your personal belongings the same day you leave the facility. If you come back later, you just feel bad all over again. As tempting as it may be, don't take hospital property, erase or delete computer files, or otherwise sabotage projects or people. Leaving gracefully is a skill that will last much longer than the immature antics you can do when angry. You also don't want to jeopardize any chance for good references or put yourself in a legally risky situation.

Severance pay, references, and benefit status are the most important issues to consider with a layoff. If possible, do not discuss severance at that first notification meeting. See if you can make an appointment for the next day. Delaying the discussion will give you a chance to deal with your emotions and be able to think and negotiate clearly. Document as much as you possibly can about the layoff meeting. It is acceptable to take notes, or if you cannot do so, write down everything you remember as soon as you leave the meeting.

Once you have received official notification of the reduction in force, be sure to meet with someone from the human resources department. You need to review your present benefit status and learn about unused sick time and vacation. Ask about contract issues related to layoffs if you work in a union-contract facility. If you are enrolled in retirement, deferred-compensation, or profit-sharing plans, find out about rollovers and buyout options. If you have medical benefits, get all the information you need to sign up for COBRA (Consolidated Omnibus Budget Reconciliation Act) health benefits. COBRA benefits are legislated benefits that give you the right to continue your health insurance, at your own expense, for up to 18 months after you are laid off.

Ask about outplacement assistance. Although it is usually offered only for managerial positions, you may be able to trade a lower severance package for that option. If you have outplacement help, use it, as these folks can help you develop or revise your resume, set up interviews, do a skills/job analysis, and provide other helpful resources and contacts.

Ask about references. Find out from your nurse manager and the human resources department exactly who will be providing your reference information and what will be said. Make requests about written and verbal references during the severance-negotiation meeting.

Negotiate as much severance pay as you can. The usual method of computing severance is one week for every year of service. Many managers feel guilty about layoffs, so use that to your advantage. Ask for twice as much as you think you can get. You can always back down, but you can never ask for more. If you can't get as much severance as you have earned, ask for an additional vacation/sick days payout, job counseling, or outplacement services in lieu of more severance pay.

Don't sit too long on the severance pay you have earned. The time goes quickly, and most employers want folks to have connected employment history on their resume. If you take a year off to sail to Greece, it will be an issue when you get back into the workforce. Most job searches take about three and one half months, so do not get complacent, even if you have a long-term severance package.

Apply for unemployment insurance/benefits as soon as you can. It can take a long time for the process to be completed and to get your first check. As tempting as it is to delay this step, the sooner you apply, the sooner you will have a check. Most states have a Web site so you can apply online. You will probably have a phone or in-person interview to ask about the layoff and how your benefits will pay out.

Tell everyone you know that you are looking for work. As much as you want to keep the layoff private, the word leaks out anyway. Also, keep in mind that networking with your colleagues will likely lead you to a new job. Compile a list of professional references. Never place someone on your reference list without asking his/her permission first. Include the person's name, address, phone number, and position. Submit this on a sheet of paper separate from a job application, and only when asked to do so.

Be sure to keep your resume updated. If you keep it ready to go, you can jump on any job opportunity that you hear of. You can also share copies with colleagues who may have leads. Have business cards printed. They need only have your name, address, and phone number. You can print them on your personal computer or at an office supply/printing store. If you have business cards, you can give them to people you meet so they have a way to reach you if they hear of a job you might be interested in.

Keep your interview skills polished. It never hurts to do an interview once in a while, even if you don't want to change positions. Don't make the mistake I did long ago of never interviewing and having no contact list. When I had my first layoff, I had no recruiters or resources to contact. Not a good plan! I had to start completely over again and re-create my job network from scratch. Don't make my mistake!

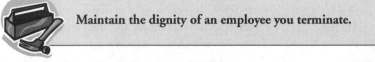

For Your Toolkit

Maintain the dignity of an employee you terminate.

During the stressful time after a layoff, take good care of yourself. Get plenty of sleep, eat healthfully, and get regular exercise. Give yourself a few days to regroup before you begin job hunting. Recovering from a layoff takes time. Be choosy about the jobs you interview for and don't take the first job you find because you are scared you won't get another offer. Do an honest self-assessment about your life, the type of job you want, and your personal and professional goals. This will allow you to find a job that is a good fit for your life. If you give yourself time to adjust and are a bit cautious about choosing a new job, you will find that your layoff turned into a blessing in disguise. They all have for me—and I have had four!

For Your Toolkit

Layoffs can be a blessing in disguise!

If You Are the Person Doing the Laying Off

It is a gut-wrenching experience to downsize staff positions. If you are the nurse manager or executive notifying others of eliminated positions, you have additional stress during this time. Keep in mind that there are two sets of people affected by the layoff decision. Those who stay and those who go. People that leave the organization through layoffs are called the layoff victims. Those who are left in the organization are the layoff survivors. Often, the survivors have as many issues as (if not more than) the victims.

Layoff survivors usually become cynical and have a loss of confidence and trust in management. They feel decreased loyalty and very low morale. They tend to work harder, but not smarter, in efforts to support their survivor guilt. They may have ambiguity and feel sad that folks left, but glad they still have a job. There is increased stress, decreased productivity, increased costs and overtime, and changed workflows.

People who survive a layoff can feel these emotions:

- Fear
- Anger
- Defensiveness
- Sense of betrayal
- Sense of entitlement
- Inflexibility
- Militancy/union activism
- An "us versus them" mentality
- Victimization
- Denial/ostrich syndrome
- Perception of powerlessness
- Tunnel vision

It is critical to manage a layoff kindly and effectively. The backlash to one handled poorly will last for years. Maintain the dignity of both the layoff victims and the survivors. Look at alternatives to layoffs, including voluntary retirement, pay freezes, full-time status changed to part-time, etc. Be able to speak to these efforts with the layoff survivors.

Layoff interventions must be planned and implemented prior to the layoffs and immediately after they occur. Denial that layoff interventions are required often leads managers to deny that there are problems with the survivors. This denial makes the healing process harder to accomplish. Don't get trapped in the idea that keeping layoffs secret is a good plan. The longer the advance notification of a layoff is, the better employees can face and manage anxiety. Ethics also plays a part here. Advance notice is almost always helpful. It is neither kind nor ethical to withhold notice for other than strictly legal reasons.

The most important tools to manage a layoff are education and communication. Recovery from a layoff must be managed from the top, using your time and coaching skills. Be empathetic and patient. Allow, accept, and encourage venting. Anticipate that survivors will make mistakes. Allow the survivors time to rebuild trust and deal with their grief (Marks, 1994). By being proactive and empathetic, you can seize the opportunity to improve organizational results over the long term.

For Your Toolkit

> **The most important tools to manage a layoff are education and communication.**

If you are doing layoffs and remaining in the facility, remember these tips:

- Communication is not just important; it is everything.
- Flood the survivors with information in all forms—oral, written, informal, formal, verbal, and nonverbal.
- Use open communication, not controlled or contrived.
- Tell the truth.
- Never say "never."
- Survivors will be shell-shocked and searching for control.
- Employees will need assurance, consistency, and continuity.
- Explain the rationale for layoff and selection strategies.
- Be visible as a manager on all your units and in areas of responsibility.
- Be empathetic and share feelings.
- Be authentic, not controlled or worried about "image."
- Identify the caretaking services offered to layoff victims—severance, outplacement, etc., and talk about them with layoff survivors.
- Lead with your heart first, then your head.
- Remember, managing a layoff is more like managing a funeral than a financial situation.
- Maintain the dignity of both victims and survivors.

If You Are Terminated

Termination is traumatic no matter how or why it happens. Sometimes it is totally unexpected. Usually termination results from an employee's having ongoing difficulties in a workplace. Counseling and clarification of work objectives have usually occurred at least once, and often several times. Most terminations occur after several counseling meetings and after all other options to resolve the performance have been attempted. Rarely does a termination occur immediately. This only happens when significant policy or legal violations have occurred. Most facilities have employee handbooks that outline the circumstances of immediate termination. Be sure you review and are familiar with what actions constitute immediate termination.

Being terminated from your position usually means you will not receive any severance pay. You will likely receive all earned sick and vacation time in your final check. Usually the check is presented to you at the time of termination. You are usually escorted from the building. Most managers try to do terminations away from the unit so employees do not have to be escorted through the unit or past their colleagues. This doesn't always happen smoothly, however.

Turner Layoff Checklist

1. Don't panic.

2. Remember, this is not a disciplinary action.

3. Don't get angry with your supervisor or the person who tells you.

4. Don't discuss severance at the first meeting. If possible, reschedule when you are not in shock.

5. Create a resume and keep it up to date.

6. Document as much as you can about your layoff meeting. Take notes during the meeting or write all you can remember as soon as you leave the meeting.

7. Meet with a human resources representative to review your current benefit status and sign up for COBRA.

8. Ask for outplacement service, especially in lieu of severance.

9. Negotiate hard for severance pay. The rule of thumb is one week per year of service. However, most human resources managers feel guilty about layoffs, so use this to your advantage. Ask for twice what you think you can get.

10. Don't sit on your severance money as though it will last forever.

11. Clarify that your employer reference will document your departure as a reduction in force (RIF), not a termination.

12. Apply quickly for unemployment; it takes time to activate.

(continues)

Turner Layoff Checklist (continued)

13. Leave the same day and take all your belongings. It is too painful to come back later.

14. Don't take hospital property or erase computer files. It may harm your chances of a good reference later on.

15. Ask for written references from human resources and your supervisor.

16. Keep an updated list of professional references.

17. Tell *everyone* you are looking for a job.

18. Keep in contact with colleagues.

19. Do not burn your bridges by publicly complaining about your previous employer. You never know who is sitting behind you in a restaurant or is in the next bathroom stall!

20. Take special care of yourself and try to use what you have the most of: time!

21. Review books and articles on resume writing, interviewing, and career choices.

22. Remember: you are not what you do!

Adapted from *American Association of Critical Care Nurses Transitions in Healthcare* curricula, 1996. Original Source. © 1994 Turner Healthcare Associates.

The usual termination process involves a confidential meeting between you, your manager, and a representative from human resources. If you are in a bargaining unit and represented by a union, you have the right to have a union representative at the meeting. A termination document is prepared and reviewed. The reasons for your termination should be clearly identified to you, including what policies or procedures were broached. You will be asked to sign the document and receive a copy. Keep in mind that signing the document does not imply agreement with the circumstances, only receipt of the document. If there is a grievance procedure, it should be reviewed at that time. If the manager or human resources person does not review that procedure, ask to have it discussed. You will be asked to turn in your badge, keys, or other electronic entry or documentation devices. If you have an office, you will likely be escorted to the office and asked to pack your personal items. You will not be allowed to retrieve files, data, or employee contact information. If you have a locker, you will be asked to clean it out with a witness present. Take everything with you, as it will be difficult to return. Some facilities will not allow you to re-enter the facility unless you are a patient seeking care. Once you complete packing your personal items, you will be escorted to your vehicle. You may be escorted off the property as well while you are driving out of the parking lot.

Being terminated from a position is a traumatic event. As tempting as it is to lash out at your manager, staff, or human resources staff—*don't*. This can harm your chance for a good reference as well as burn bridges for you in the future. Stay as quiet and emotionally neutral as you can. Save your tears, hurt, and anger for a private location. Those are normal reactions to termination, so don't feel like you are overreacting. No matter what the circumstances, termination feels personal, and many unpleasant feelings come up after it occurs.

It is likely you will be contacted by co-workers. Most managers downplay the termination of a staff member and are mandated not to divulge any of the details to other staff on the unit. However, if the circumstances of the termination involved co-worker witnesses, there will be many different versions circulating about what actually took place. When you are contacted by co-workers, try hard not to badmouth everyone and all that happened. Of course, you can talk candidly to your trusted friends, but be careful what you say if your close friends are also your co-workers.

You may want to brainstorm with a trusted friend to come up with a couple of summary sentences that you can say whenever anyone calls you. That way you don't have to relive the pain of the incident every time you pick up the phone. Consider having your voicemail or answering machine pick up calls until you feel emotionally able to talk with people. If the situation involves the news media and you are contacted, *do not (!)* make any statements that can be perceived as slanderous. Although it is tempting to let loose with a news reporter and say everything you didn't get to say to your manager, it is a bad idea. Remember, *nothing* is ever off the record with any kind of reporter. If you are unable to remain neutral while discussing the circumstances, have a trusted friend, spouse, or attorney read a statement on your behalf. Avoid writing letters to a newspaper, hospital administration, or board of directors complaining about your termination. You want to keep your dignity as much as possible.

Maintain your personal cool and wait until some time passes—even a few days can make a huge difference. If you have a potential legal case, contact a lawyer directly and do not talk to your colleagues about any possibility of legal action. It will complicate the situation later on. Do apply for unemployment insurance quickly, although in many cases of termination, you will not be eligible. Since the eligibility criteria vary from state to state and are confusing, go ahead and apply. You may end up being eligible for payments, and it takes several weeks to get the process in place. Most states allow you to apply online.

Most employee terminations are related to poor performance or violation of company policy. Even if you don't agree, most people are usually clear about why you were terminated. Sometimes the reasons for your termination may have nothing to do with you. It may be related to a reorganization, a new administrative team, or a new corporate direction. It is difficult to separate your performance from yourself, but the reality is that you are not what you do. Try not to personalize the termination as an insult to you as a person, because it will delay your ability to move out of the bitterness and hurt of the situation and into a new role.

I routinely hear on the Monster.com message board from healthcare workers who have been terminated. The question most frequently asked is how to deal with the termination on interviews and job applications. Many of these folks want to lie or leave out information about their termination. It is my belief that trying to hide a termination or lie about it is a bad idea. The healthcare industry is too incestuous and everyone knows everybody, so you can never remain anonymous. You may end up having to work in a new job with someone who knows what happened. I think your best policy is to be up front about the reason for the termination and what you have learned from the situation. It shows maturity and acknowledgment of your accountability for your actions. If your termination has legal ramifications or you are placed in a chemical diversion program, be honest about that as well.

For Your Toolkit

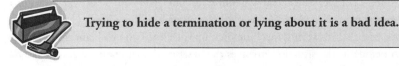

Trying to hide a termination or lying about it is a bad idea.

It is not easy to do, but keep in mind that rumors circulate and sometimes they can be worse than the actual circumstances. Legal cases will become public record and knowledge at some point—even years later—so you don't want any unplanned surprises. In my experience, employees who are honest about their mistakes and talk about what they learned from the termination do the best with moving into new roles.

The other thing to remember is that people tend not to talk about terminations that have happened in the past. Being terminated is a lot like being married to an alcoholic. You think that you are the only person you know in that situation until you mention it to someone. Then you find out that they had the same experience. There are lots of people (and nurses) out there who have been terminated from a job, even though you don't always hear about it.

You can be terminated from a position and still be successful. I am living proof of that. I was terminated from a position as a unit clerk while I was in nursing school. While I still dispute the appropriateness and rationale for the termination after all these years, I maintained my dignity during the process. I found a new job, and learned a lot (not all of it pleasant!) from the experience.

If You Terminate an Employee

If you are in a management role and must terminate an employee, there are a few things to keep in mind. First of all, be kind and compassionate. Being terminated is a humiliating experience. No matter how angry you are at the employee for the incredibly stupid thing he or she did to get fired, don't communicate that with your body language or words.

For Your Toolkit

Be kind and compassionate if you are terminating an employee.

Pick a confidential and private location to talk with the employee being terminated. Close your office door. If people can hear the conversation through the door, consider using a conference room away from the unit. If the employee is to be escorted out of the unit, obtain the employee's personal belongings yourself, if possible. It is very difficult for an employee to walk past co-workers after just being terminated. Save them that loss of dignity.

If you must share the vacancy of the position, do not state that the employee was terminated in your communication with staff. Use ambiguous phrases like "left to pursue other opportunities" or "decided to try something new" to explain the vacancy. Do not discuss the reasons or the circumstances about the termination with any employees other than human resources staff or supervisors who need to be made aware. Confidentiality is crucial, not only for the dignity of the employee, but for legal purposes. Although terminating an employee is never easy, it is something that will affect the person for a long time. Be gentle and sincere. Your employee will be grateful—and you may avoid a lawsuit. Besides, you never know what might happen. Hopefully, you are never terminated from your position. But if that takes place, you would want to be treated kindly with dignity and compassion as well.

Resignation

At some point in your career, you will want to change jobs. You may want to leave the facility or simply move to another unit. You can resign and keep work relationships intact with just a little bit of proactive planning. Determine your date for resignation first. Consult your facility employee handbook for the required resignation notice time frames. The usual rule of thumb is two weeks' notice for a staff position and four weeks' notice for a management position. Don't leave without any warning. You could be reported to your state board of nursing for patient abandonment.

Resignations should be made in writing; however, leaving the letter for your manager to find on his/her desk is a last resort. Make an appointment with your manager to discuss your resignation. Explain your reasons briefly, e.g., you want to learn new skills or try something new. Do not use the meeting to complain about your co-workers or the manager. State the last day you will be working. Managers appreciate it if you resign at the end of a payroll or scheduling cycle. Sometimes that isn't possible, but it makes the resignation smoother.

Inform your manager *before* you tell your co-workers. It is very frustrating as a manager to hear about a resignation through the grapevine, and it is disrespectful of the manager. You will likely be asked by your manager to sign at least one document for human resources that is part of the resignation paperwork. Keep a copy of the document and of your resignation letter. If you are unhappy on the unit where you are currently working, do not use your last few days to complain about your co-workers or the workload. Finish out your shifts and maintain your dignity.

For Your Toolkit

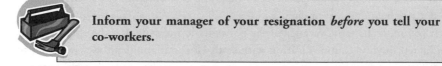

Inform your manager of your resignation *before* you tell your co-workers.

If you transfer out of a unit but are not leaving the facility, you usually don't need to resign formally. Most facilities have a transfer document that can be completed and

Turner Termination Checklist

1. Don't panic!

2. Don't get angry with your supervisor or the person who tells you of the termination.

3. Create a resume and keep it up to date.

4. Document as much as you can about your termination meeting. Take notes during the meeting or write all you can remember as soon as you leave the meeting. Keep copies of all materials you sign or receive.

5. If someone from human resources is not present at the termination meeting, ask to meet with someone to review your current benefit status, and sign up for COBRA *before* you leave the building.

6. Clarify what specific reference information will be provided to prospective employers.

7. Apply quickly for unemployment. You may not be eligible, but if you are, it takes time to activate.

8. Leave the same day and take all your belongings. It is too painful to come back later.

9. Don't take hospital property or erase computer files. It may harm your chances of a good reference later on.

10. Keep an updated list of professional references.

11. Tell everyone you are looking for a job. You can do this without divulging the termination.

(continues)

Turner Termination Checklist (continued)

12. Decide if you want to keep in contact with colleagues.

13. Do not burn your bridges by publicly complaining about your previous employer. You never know who is sitting behind you in a restaurant or is in the next bathroom stall!

14. Take special care of yourself and try to use what you have the most of: *time!*

15. Consider journaling about your termination experience. You can learn a lot from putting your experiences in writing.

16. Remember: you are not what you do!

Turner Healthcare Associates, Inc., © 2005.

turned into your manager or the human resources department. This means you change units but do not resign from the facility. If you are transferring, meet with your current manager to let him/her know you are going to interview for a position on another unit. Chances are they will hear about your interest in a transfer from the manager who interviewed you anyway. It is professional behavior to tell your current manager where you are interested in transferring and why. Keep your comments brief and about your professional development. Don't talk about how frustrated you are or how much you hate working with so and so. It is better to describe your reasons for transferring in terms of your own goals, e.g., learn new skills, meet new people, go back to school. Your manager may ask you to stay longer on the unit than you wish in order to accommodate staffing. Most facilities have transfer deadlines and expect current managers and future managers to negotiate a transfer plan together. Do your best to be flexible and honor both managers' needs to have you working, if you can.

If a going-away gathering is an option, participate graciously in the planning. If you do not want a gathering, say so early, so it doesn't appear that you are raining on your co-workers' parade. Many staff like to have farewell events, as it is a formal method to initiate the transition process. Whatever you decide, be gracious and kind to the co-workers you are leaving behind.

Negotiating a Raise

Many nurses believe their workload has increased dramatically, and that they are long overdue for a raise. Although the national shortage of nurses has caused salaries to rise significantly, there is still room for salary growth in most positions.

Before you ask your boss for a raise, do your homework. Assess your performance from your supervisor's perspective. What is the most important thing you do for him/her? Would s/he hire you today? What does s/he consider your talents to be? How does s/he think you can improve your performance? Once you have these potential answers in your mind, you are ready to meet with him/her.

After you have created a clear idea of how you are making your boss's life easier, schedule a meeting and present your case. Use a percentage, not a dollar figure, when voicing your raise request. In 2005, the national average for raises was 3.7% (Bach, 2005). In the best outcome, your case will be clearly stated and your boss will agree to a raise.

If your raise is denied, be sure to say thanks anyway, and thank your boss for listening. Don't leave angry or make threats about resigning your position. Ask your boss for specifics on what you can do to be successful in getting a raise in the future. Even if you disagree with your boss, listen to the information. If the feedback is mostly negative, then you may want to polish your resume. You don't want to stay in a dead-end job or end up feeling unappreciated. Either one can be a big career mistake.

Professional Malaise

One day it just happens. You get to work and feel that what you are doing just doesn't matter anymore. You wonder, "What else can I do to make a difference?" Several more shifts go by and you feel unmotivated and stuck in a rut. You may be unsure what to do next and decide it is about the difficult tasks nurses do for patients and a lousy workplace environment. You don't readily seek change because it is uncomfortable. Some people call this "burnout." Burnout implies inability to change the circumstances of your work perceptions. I prefer the term "professional malaise" because I believe the situation can be adjusted. Nurses with professional malaise use more sick days, are less productive, are depressed, and often talk about how miserable they are. Their circumstances don't change, and many leave bedside care or the profession of nursing altogether. There are many responsibilities that nurses have today at work, as well as the stress that goes with them. Because of this it is easy to understand why so many nurses suffer from burnout. To avoid this, you must care for the caregiver, just as you care for the patient.

Nurses with burnout are easy to spot. They are tired, crabby, and usually surly if they have a student or preceptee. They often get sluggish halfway through a shift or

Symptoms of professional malaise

- You feel no accountability toward the profession of nursing.
- Experienced nurses don't help you.
- Other disciplines encroach or dump.
- No one understands bedside nursing care.
- You feel powerless and inflexible.
- You feel unable to deal with work-related conflicts.
- You're not sure you are in an organization that represents you.
- You hate intraprofessional infighting.
- You have no strategic plan or vision for yourself or the nursing profession.

speak of longing to be somewhere other than where they are. They get irritable with an unexpected challenge or if a new grad asks the same question more than once (Brzezicki, 2005).

Nurses with the burnout blues, as Lisa Brzezicki describes them, fail to recognize how burnout symptoms affect their overall physical health. Nurses are so busy taking care of others that they often neglect to take care of themselves. Nurses often fail to get their cholesterol checked, to lose weight, to quit smoking, or to exercise more. How many of you are in your late 50s and still don't have enough time to take the screening colonoscopy recommended for everyone when they turn 50?

Hospitals are starting to provide health programs for nurses right in the workplace with smoking-cessation and weight-loss programs or in-house yoga experts. These kinds of programs are great sources for healthier lifestyles, but the ultimate choice to take better care of yourself rests with you. What have you done for yourself lately? It may be something as simple as taking a quiet moment to enjoy music or a cup of coffee. It might be walking the dog, playing golf, reading a book, or taking a nap. Whatever it is, be sure to unwind, relax, and reenergize. Make sure you make time for yourself in your schedule. You deserve it, and you will be able to look at your nursing future with excitement instead of dread.

There is nothing wrong or unusual about having professional malaise. Many nurses have the feelings described above at least once during their careers. The difference between those who stay in nursing and those who leave the profession has to do with personal headspace. Professional malaise can be embraced and resolved.

There are numerous reasons for developing professional malaise. You don't believe you have individual accountability toward the profession of nursing. You feel that the more experienced nurses don't help you to learn or excel. They get angry when you ask questions, make a mistake, or take longer than they do to do a task. You may perceive other disciplines either encroaching on your areas of responsibility or dumping their tasks on you. You feel that no one understands what you go through giving bedside nursing care every day, and that no one wants to know the challenges of your role. You feel powerless and inflexible. You feel unable to deal with work-related conflicts and the smallest incident or issue sends you over the edge and off the deep end.

You begin to wonder about the leadership in your institution and you're not sure you have an organization that represents your professional perspective. You feel that the nurses you work with fight too much among themselves about issues within the profession and do nothing to resolve them. You feel that there is no strategic planning or vision for you or the nursing profession, and that nothing will change.

Any or all of these feelings and perceptions can be indications of professional malaise. If you have one or more of them, you are not alone. Professional malaise is not a death sentence for your nursing career. With recognition, support, and an individual place to change your headspace, you can move through professional malaise. You will come out of the experience as a better nurse because of it.

Solutions for Professional Malaise

There are ways to combat professional malaise. It means being honest about having professional malaise in the first place and creating a method to deal with it. You need to make changes in your perceptions and in your work life. This doesn't always mean that everyone around you will behave differently. What changes about the situation is in your personal headspace. Dealing with professional malaise doesn't necessarily mean you have to change jobs. However, it does mean that you need to make changes in your work life. The changes will likely have profound effects on your state of professional malaise but may be difficult to manage.

The most important first step is to identify the problem. If you are unclear as to what actually is the problem, try taking the career assessment identified in this book. Once you pinpoint why you are feeling lousy, you can fix the right problem. Your professional malaise may extend if you fix the wrong problem, so it is worthwhile to take the time to evaluate the root cause of your discomfort.

For Your Toolkit

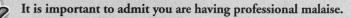

It is important to admit you are having professional malaise.

Taking action to identify the right problem means you will need to look at where you are currently in your career, as well as where you need to be for the future. It may mean considering educational or professional development to improve your opportunities and options. Most importantly, create a new attitude. This means no more whining. If you whine, you are a victim. If you are a victim, you will feel powerless and perceive that you can do nothing to change your circumstances. Nothing is further from the truth.

By addressing your professional malaise and the cause(s) of it, you will begin a personal journey. You will evaluate your future as a nurse and create a plan to implement self-marketing strategies. The journey will likely involve conflict management, but you will need that to enhance resolution. During professional malaise, it can also help to find a mentor and/or a coach. This coach or mentor can help you identify the root cause of your professional malaise, deal with the changes needed to get you out of professional malaise, and help you create your personal plan.

Coping with Transition: Change Your Headspace

"It is easy to come up with new ideas: the hard part is letting go of what worked for you two years ago, but will soon be out of date"

—PAUL GANN

Nurses routinely deal with transition. Changes happen in health care and nursing practice all the time. Changing policies, procedures, patients, and regulations are everywhere, no matter in what kind of nursing environment you work. It is difficult to deal with the emotional upheaval and moral angst included in such changes.

Mitchell Marks (1994) highlights the change process that organizations must go through to be successful and deal with transition. That process can be extrapolated to individual nurses as well. Nurses tend to become militant and defensive if they perceive that organizational changes in a facility are negative. This negativity applies to personal changes as well. Nurses are great patient advocates, but not particularly good at advocating for themselves in a positive way.

Marks identifies two types of transition: event-driven and planned transformation. Event-driven transition is triggered by an event, such as a merger, organizational redesign, or downsizing. Planned transformation is a large-scale culture change consisting of a cumulative series of changes that signal transition from an old way to new way of operating (Marks, 1994). The nursing profession was exposed to both types of transition during the restructuring and redesign sagas of the 1990s. Individual nurses experience planned transition every time a process or procedural change is made in a healthcare organization. Nurses also experience event transition when a facility is merged or sold.

In addition to the industry-wide transition issues that have happened in health care over the past two decades (managed care, prospective payment, work restructuring and redesign, patient safety mandates), there are numerous intraprofessional nursing issues that have never been resolved, e.g., What is the most appropriate level for entry into nursing practice, ADN or BSN? Which organization is the one professional voice for nursing?

On top of all that, there is also an accelerated nursing care expectation. Completing the same number of patient care tasks in a significantly shorter time frame causes frustration for nursing staff because they believe they cannot offer the same quality of care in a shortened time span. This emphasis on time ignores the fact that healing takes its own time, differs with each patient, and cannot be regulated. It leads to nursing based on task completion instead of caring for the patient as a whole person. The resulting chaos has caused several states to legislate minimum safe staffing regulations and ratios.

For Your Toolkit

> **The emphasis on time leads to nursing based on task completion instead of caring for the patient as a whole person.**

There are several stages that Marks (1994) identifies that each nurse goes through when dealing with change:

- Stage 1 = shock and fear.
- Stage 2 = defensive retreat.
- Stage 3 = acknowledgment of need for change.
- Stage 4 = adaptation to change.

These stages are similar to the three stages of change outlined by Edwin Lewin (Robbins, 1996):

- Unfreezing = assessment of current environment and issues followed by shock and fear (this is where transition occurs).
- Changing = demonstrating new behaviors.
- Refreezing = new behaviors become routine and the norm.

Lewin believes that there are forces for and against change working at the same time. This is part of the reason nurses feel ambivalent about change, both personally and professionally. If you are going to make changes, you must go through a transition process before actually making the changes.

It is common to resist change. Organizational change in health care is caused by technology, knowledge, consumer demands, resource availability, and social attitudes. This leaves lots of opportunity for resistance to change, caused by:

- employee attitudes and work habits.
- anxiety.
- cohesiveness.
- organizational rigidity—inflexibility, controls, rules, and policies.
- lack of trust and questioning the motives of others.
- too much confidence in past ways of doing things.
- job security.

It is also common for people to fear their own empowerment, which often represents change. According to Caroline Myss (2003), change signals a loss of control and entry into the unknown. She believes that even beyond the fear of change, empowerment represents isolation, which most people will do anything to avoid. This becomes a paradoxical view of empowerment. Rick Warren (2002) writes that there is no growth without change, no change without fear or loss, and no loss without pain.

For Your Toolkit

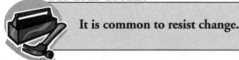

It is common to resist change.

Managing change uses organizational development skills based on the idea that organizations consist of building blocks. Those building blocks are groups and teams. Organizations require collaboration, not competition between groups. Groups should lead decision-making because they are the source of information. Organizations, groups, and individuals manage affairs according to goals, not controls. Individuals and groups must participate in planning and implementing change. They will support what they help create.

Managing change begins with assessment to determine how to proceed. The manager's job is to help staff deal with change. Managers may need help and training to deal with change, just like employees. Your job is to help yourself and colleagues deal with change. Your role in facilitating a positive change process includes being an educator, communicator, participant, facilitator, supporter, negotiator, and influencer.

When a nurse deals with change, there are tasks that s/he must perform for personal change to be implemented effectively. It is normal for any type of change to cause conflict, fear, confusion, and an urge to return to the old way of doing things. Conflict-management skills are necessary during the change process, whether the change is personal or professional. Effective communication skills are vital so that others understand what you are doing. It is important to keep everyone supporting you in the feedback loop. Here are some tips to deal with the unsettling feelings of transition:

- Get educated about the changes and what is necessary to make them.
- Communicate with your personal support system.
- Participate actively in the changes you are making (you are not a victim).
- Stand firm in your desire to change even when those around you question it.
- Negotiate conflicts that arise from your changes.

It is important to remember that you can't have change without some sort of transition. You can change your personal perspectives and headspace much like a healthcare organization can change its culture of performance. When you change your headspace you can:

- create a new personal structure of priorities and philosophy.
- manage personal stress and recovery through implementing changes and using the refreezing process.
- help yourself be successful.
- create new personal opportunities.

For Your Toolkit

You can't have change without transition.

You may find yourself initially resisting a new headspace and professional philosophy. You may challenge new perspectives by creating dysfunctional behaviors for yourself. You may see yourself doing things as coping strategies that are really personal sabotage:

- Resisting personal change.
- Regressive behaviors—compulsive eating, arguing, and bickering with co-workers or family members.
- Feeling powerless or victimized.
- Feeling totally unmotivated.
- Using "crisis du jour" strategies to avoid making changes because you don't have time to really change anything.

- Constricted communications.
- Using outmoded or unsuccessful personal systems for success.
- Unable to do things differently because there are no others to offer a consensus for your choices.
- Not allocating resources (time, energy, money, passion) to the changes you wish to make.
- Making a programmatic, flavor-of-the-month change instead of a philosophic one, often why dieters fail to lose weight.

Career difficulties are an invitation for you to make changes. Transition can become a new way of life. Managing transition is essential for a successful career-related change experience. Transition management is important in dealing with changes in your personal life as well. Recovery from the transition is essential to the process and means you must deal with the emotional realities of the transition. Going through transition is equivalent to the unfreezing step outlined in Lewin's change theory.

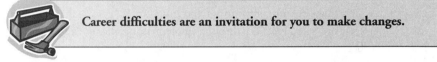

For Your Toolkit

Career difficulties are an invitation for you to make changes.

Keep in mind that all professional transitions are opportunities for you to do things differently. If you are in a career transition, here are some tips to get through it:

- Conduct a job self-analysis/skills inventory using some of the tools in this book.
- Define the product—you! Evaluate your resume, interview skills, and self-presentation.
- Pay attention to your intuition. It will affect your career success.
- Get the word out about your interests and roles.
- Don't go for the quick fix.
- Don't delegate or defer your career work.
- *Remember: who you are is not what you do!*

Recovery After Transition

There is no magic recipe for dealing with personal change and transition. Transition is a steady and constant state in health care these days. Transition is usually not a fun experience, but it is necessary for personal and career growth. After surviving a transition, just about everyone sees it as a growth experience. Every major event in your life (graduation, first job, marriage, children, divorce, and death) has personal transition as a part of the experience. No one can escape dealing with transition. However, you can determine how you deal with it.

According to Marks (1994), people change either by design or default. This means that you can change your approach to transition by purposefully creating strategies or you can do nothing and go with whatever happens. Nurses tend to go with what they know. Familiarity is comfortable but not always effective. If you want to do things differently, you need to change your plan for reacting to change.

For Your Toolkit

No one can escape dealing with transition.

Experiencing transition by itself will not alter your existing mental model about what is changing. There are several ways to move through transition. You can retain old attitudes and change no behaviors, *or* you can alter your mental model and settle into attitudes and behaviors inadvertently reinforced during your transition process, *or* you can alter your mental model and rely on attitudes and behaviors reinforced by the design of your personal transition-management strategy. It's up to you to decide how you want to move through transition. But remember, change and transition will happen no matter what you do.

For Your Toolkit

People change by design or default.

If you decide to manage your transition, you can link your recovery plan to a personal quality-improvement process:

- Identify what you want and how to get it.
- Draft a personal recovery plan.
- Identify the essential work you must do to maintain your personal performance standards.
- Determine creative approaches to continuing the essential work you must do personally and professionally.
- Focus on minimizing fear and conflict.
- Create your own personal context for transition recovery by creating your own new personal structure and philosophy.
- Aim high and don't take the easy way out.

- Create a new personal vision for yourself, using the tools in this book, and accept that there is no alternative.
- Accept responsibility for your personal failures and create your future success.

If you do not create a personal plan for change outlining the changes you wish to embrace, you will resort to doing what you know—going with the old behaviors. Reject the temptation to create a flavor-of-the-month change. It doesn't work in organizations and it won't work personally. In the absences of a plan, people go with what they know. To survive and thrive during transition, try these strategies:

- Link your self-assessments to your career development plan.
- Draft a written personal recovery plan.
- Rebuild your spirit.
- Create your own context for recovery.
- Use proactive venting and encourage others to use it as well.
- Focus on the work you are doing to transition, not the process.
- Create a new personal process, not a flavor-of-the-month program.
- Provide yourself with resources (stress reduction, time alone, exercise).
- Say over and over what you want to change.
- Motivate from the top down: first your head, then your heart.
- Motivate from the inside—persuasion of your heart and mind, not just doing the behaviors.
- Be patient and empathetic with yourself and your resistance. This is *hard* work!
- Remember that professional recovery and transition are personal imperatives to remain healthy and employed in a competitive (albeit fairly dysfunctional) industry.

You can create a new personal structure and philosophy by identifying your personal and professional direction. Consider writing your own mission statement for your life and career. Use the self-assessment tools in this book to determine what you need to do differently. Determine the core competencies you need for successful transition, e.g., time management, exercise, learning to say "no." Create a contract with yourself for the changes you are making. This will force you to decide what kind of personal and professional culture you need to be immersed in to be successful with your transition plan. Minimize contact with individuals and organizations who will not encourage your success. Determine how you will fit your job around your life instead of your life around your job. You can create your own life design and architecture you need to be successful, such as joining a gym, hiring a gardener, or engaging in spiritual practices.

You can revitalize yourself after the changes you have made take place. It is important to understand that you need to recover from the transition process after you have implemented your personal changes. Revitalize from the top down. First change your headspace, then your heart. Now it is time to align your personal and professional work with your new personal order and priorities. If needed, work on rebuilding trust within yourself and with co-workers. These strategies allow you to walk your walk and talk your talk.

You have opportunities in this new personal structure and philosophy. You can resuscitate your spirit—something rarely achieved without transition. Malaise recovery and revitalization mean renewing your personal resources, enhancing your personal and professional work methods and boundaries, and living your personal vision for yourself and your life. You can embrace personal and professional lifelong learning and share your strategies with others when embracing proactive transition management.

For Your Toolkit

Malaise recovery and revitalization mean renewing your personal resources, enhancing your personal and professional work methods and boundaries, and living your personal vision for yourself and your life.

Mastering Career Change

You can master career change. According to numerous experts, the average person changes jobs six to eight times in a lifetime. This can happen as a matter of choice or involuntarily. Some folks leave jobs involuntarily because the job is being eliminated or because of poor performance. Others move to other organizations because their job was a bad fit or they were disillusioned with the organization.

Most people do not understand the skills required for surviving a career change. Personal characteristics and qualities to thrive, not just survive, include energy and self-direction, self-confidence, commitment to a long-term strategy, problem-solving ability, an understanding of how to use career resources, and the ability to use wisely the positive and negative feedback you receive.

You can survive and thrive during a job change. It takes developing your problem-solving skills and refining and reframing your thinking. You are always more employable if you have a constant attitude of being willing to learn. Remember you are selling a product—*you!* Think of yourself as a valuable resource. While counselors and coaches can share ideas of how to be successful, only you can walk the walk. Assess your competencies, your skills, and your resume. Choose your career goals and action steps and implement your strategies to guarantee success.

Proactive Personal Transition Management

P = Prepare yourself for a high level of activity.

R = Rally yourself with a vision of a better you.

O = Offer yourself transition training by learning how to deal with transition.

A = Acknowledge your uncertainty and concerns.

C = Communicate your plans and actions to others around you so they can support you.

T = Tell others as much as you can about your transition management process.

I = Involve others in managing your transition.

V = Visit with mentors and coaches.

E = Establish your personal safety net (self-care, balanced life, career planning).

Adapted from Marks (1994). © 2001 Turner Healthcare Associates, Inc.

Turner Career Transition Model

When I completed my doctoral degree in business administration in 1998, I wrote my dissertation on the effects of restructuring clinical nursing care. I evaluated nurses' perceptions, behaviors, characteristics, and feelings about hospital restructuring of nursing departments. In the process of completing this dissertation, I created a restructuring model for organizations called the Turner Reengineering Model. While preparing the manuscript that evolved into this book, I realized that this organizational model also related to the same issues that individuals go through during transition. I revised my reengineering model to create the Turner Career Transition Model© (see Figure 8-1). I believe this is the process that every nurse making a change should use for a successful career transition.

When you experience a career transition, you always start with deciding that a change needs to be made. Once you make that decision, determine the components of actually making the change.

- What tasks do you need to complete?
- What training do you need to obtain?
- Will you relocate? Change jobs?
- How will you manage the process of getting to another place in your career?

You must deal with the emotional realities of the change you are pursuing. Most people skip this step and become overwhelmed during the change process. You need to

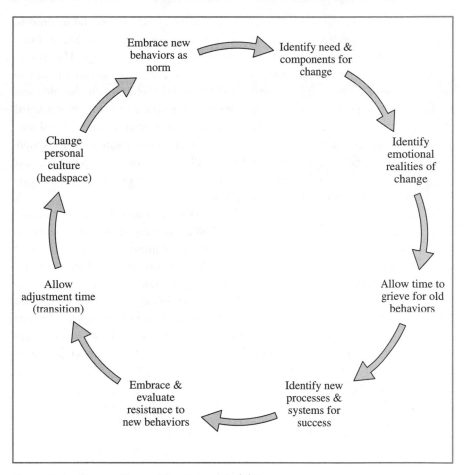

Figure 8-1   Turner Career Transition Model©
Turner Healthcare Associates, Inc. © 1998.

allow yourself to recognize sadness or attachment, to get excited about new things—whatever emotions you have about your transition. Then take some grieving time for yourself. No matter how much you want to change, you will have sadness for what will no longer be. Allow yourself grieving time. Then you will be prepared to take the steps to plan your transition and move ahead. If you don't deal with the emotional realities or do any grieving, you may remain stuck in the same spot for a long time or be overwhelmed when you do make a change.

You are now ready to move on to identifying the processes and systems you need to put in place to make the change. Do you need day care? Do you need to enroll in school? Request a transfer to another unit? Decide what you need to do and how you will do it. Determine who can help you and who will be your coaches and mentors in this process. Evaluate any resistance you have to creating these plans. Many times, individuals feel resistance and decide that it is not a good time to change. That is usually not the reason for feeling resistance. Resistance to change is caused by failing to grieve and deal with the emotional realities of leaving old behaviors. It also indicates failing to create a good plan to make the transition. Resistance isn't bad—it is a signal that you may have forgotten one or more steps in the transition process, or you may be making a change you are not ready to make. Sometimes we create a change simply to do something different but are not emotionally or spiritually prepared for that change. Don't ignore your feelings of resistance. Explore them so you can determine the underlying causes for the feelings and address them.

Once you have embraced and created the change you designed, allow yourself some adjustment time. It takes a minimum of 30 days to adjust to a new routine or process. Be gentle with yourself if you stumble at the beginning. This time becomes valuable and allows you to adapt more easily to the transition process. Once you have embraced the transition, you can begin embracing the new change as a way of life. This also means you will change your headspace into thinking that the behavior norm is the new way you are now doing things. Once you are comfortable with the new norm, you have completed the transition process. We make numerous small transitions every day, so taking time with the big changes lets us prepare and engage more completely in the change process.

Chapter 9
Your Evolving Career

Professional Nursing Roles

The professional registered nurse fulfills five specific roles within the scope of practice of registered nursing, according to the American Association of Colleges of Nursing (Turner, 1998). It is important to know what those roles include when evaluating and enhancing your career.

- Patient care provider—demonstrates skills in assessment, communication, and the provision of therapeutic nursing interventions. Uses the nursing process to develop, implement, and evaluate a plan of care.
- Teacher—demonstrates knowledge of basic principles of the teaching–learning process. Identifies clients' learning needs, capabilities, and limitations, selection of appropriate information, material, and strategies. Evaluates clients' learning outcomes.
- Advocate—states clients' rights and responsibilities as healthcare consumers, and identifies the congruence/incongruence between the clients and provider's perceptions of healthcare needs. Participates in client-care conferences communicating clients' needs.
- Professional—demonstrates knowledge of the standards of competent performance and scope of professional nursing practice. Accesses own capabilities and limitations,

and accepts accountability for actions. Establishes goals for achieving professional growth.

- Supervisor—coordinates care of clients to achieve beneficial nursing care outcomes and provide cost-effective, quality-based services.

Each nurse fulfills these roles in the professional practice setting. It doesn't matter whether you work in a hospital, home health agency, school, or church. You perform these roles every day. Assess your skills and abilities in each role. What are you best at doing? Why? Which of these roles are challenges for you? Why? This will help you evaluate the skills and competencies you need to enhance and expand.

There are additional functions that every nurse must exhibit in the workplace to be successful. One is being a knowledge worker, not just a technical worker. You need to act as the choreographer of patient care by becoming a broker of services and resources. Assist your healthcare facility to achieve organizational success. Be a participant in changing the healthcare organizational culture as well as your personal headspace. Be active in managing your own personal transition as well as organizational transitions. Talk with your colleagues and friends, and use them to validate your own professional issues and behaviors. Demonstrating these kinds of behaviors will help you become indispensable at work.

Being indispensable is easier than it sounds. There are ways to make yourself stand out in your current job setting. Focus your time on enhancing your skills and improving competencies and cultivating new ones. You will improve daily and have experiences that prepare you for new and different roles in the future. As you are working on honing your skills, you will also encounter situations that are challenging, such as angry patients or co-workers.

Dealing with Angry Patients and Co-workers

If you are confronted by an angry patient or co-worker in a work setting, what should you do? It is crucial to resist the impulse to get angry. Be quiet and listen to the person. Upset people want to be heard more than anything else. Try not to plan what you are going to say back to them while they are talking. This interferes with your ability to listen. Don't jump in and answer right away; wait until they stop talking. Then wait for a few more seconds before you respond. Resist the urge to tell them that they shouldn't feel the way they do. Feelings are valid even when you don't agree. If you have made a mistake, acknowledge that you have done so, and apologize.

Other anger-management strategies include trying to dispel false beliefs about the situation. Many times anger is based on misperceptions and miscommunication. Wait until you are both calm to talk about the situation. You can then explain the situation the way you perceive it. This often goes a long way to dispel misperceptions. It is

For Your Toolkit

Remember, upset people want to be heard. Wait until they stop talking and respond calmly.

appropriate to recognize, feel, express, and accept your own anger. Try not to speak while you are angry, as you are likely to make impulsive and unkind comments.

Talk to a friend about the situation and your feelings. Sometimes it helps to role-play an interaction with a trusted colleague or friend before you meet with the co-worker. You can also use physical activity to dispel your anger. You can also try venting your anger to an inanimate object if there is no person to receive it.

Assertive Communication

Assertive communication is another important career strategy to master. Assertive communication is used for making and refusing requests, giving and receiving recognition, and giving and receiving criticism (Stern, 1990). Samples of an assertive communication style are those that describe the situation or behavior, e.g., "When you . . ." and express your reactions or feelings about it, "I feel . . . ." You would also use an assertive style to specify the change that you want to occur, e.g., "I want you to . . . ." Assertive style also allows you to identify common goals or outcomes, e.g., "If that happens, then . . . ," or, "If you do this, then . . ."

It is common to have some anxiety and fear when considering use of an assertive style of communication. If you are anxious or fearful of it, use relaxation techniques to help you prepare. Avoid self-defeating thoughts about how you think the communication exchange will occur. Use desensitization to break your fear into smaller steps to handle them. Visualization and guided imagery may also help you focus your approach. Ask for coaching from a trusted colleague or mentor and provide your own self-coaching by being patient with your anxiety.

Managing Conflict*

Power is one of the most important job skills you can use. Power is not necessarily related to position in an organization. When you have power and use it well, you can influence many events and processes in your workplace. Power is defined as the ability to control, influence, or act. Authority is defined as the legitimate power granted to

---

*Adapted from Turner, *Nurses Guide to Managed Care.*

an individual by an organization. Power is vested in a position. Leadership is the relationship between two or more people in which one influences the other toward accomplishing a goal without legitimate power (Bernard & Walsh, 1996).

For Your Toolkit

> **When you use power well, you can influence many events and processes in your workplace.**

There are several different types of power, as defined in management texts. Personal power is the ability to link the outer capacity for action with the inner capacity of reflection. Organizational power is the ability to accomplish goals through others within an organization. Executive power is the use of personal persuasion and influence to motivate others.

Legitimate power is given to individuals based on their position in an organization. Reward power is the power to provide distribution of rewards. Coercive power is the ability to administer punishment, or the opposite of reward. Expert power is earned by an individual with expert knowledge and skills in a certain area or industry. Referent power is the ability to have influence over another based on respect and admiration.

Managers need both power (all of the types) and authority to be effective. Nurses often see power as bad or negative, but it is actually a neutral force (see Table 9-1). People who feel powerless often are unable to accomplish a goal. They then resort to other methods to get what they want, such as manipulation, dishonesty, and illegal behaviors.

People with power move through different management states of being, beginning with dictatorship. Some individuals never move past being a dictator. Others move through to seduction, persuasion, role-modeling, and finally empowerment.

TABLE 9-1   Myths About Power

Myth	*Reality*
Power is bad.	Power is neutral.
Power is a goal.	Power is a means to accomplish goals.
Powerful people are ruthless.	Powerless people are ruthless.
Power can be given to others.	Power must be earned or assumed.
It is wrong or bad to want power.	Power to accomplish goals can reduce stress and frustration.

Power becomes very important in carrying out management and leadership activities. Strong leaders use all forms of power every day to accomplish goals and motivate people to assist in meeting those goals. The use of power also may cause conflict.

Conflict is inevitable in life and at work due to complex organizations, differing employee interests and needs, and change related to transition. Many nurses are not comfortable with conflict because they have had no training to deal with it. Nursing programs do not provide much training in conflict-management or conflict-resolution skills.

Conflict can make individuals and groups feel scared and powerless. Union organizers often point out how employees may feel powerless unless they are represented by a union—whether or not the employees are actually powerless. Like power, conflict is not bad. It is inherently neutral. Conflict is not personal. But people often make it into a personal situation. Conflict can be functional because it leads to discussion, investigation, and accomplishment of new goals. Excessive conflict can be dysfunctional and lead to more strife, not problem-solving.

For Your Toolkit

Conflict is not bad or personal; it is inherently neutral.

Dysfunctional organizations usually have a lot of unresolved conflict. The senior management team may not be comfortable working through conflict to create new goals and priorities. Usually, dysfunctional organizations have a minimal amount of one-way communication—from the top down. Failing to follow through on tasks and not giving positive reinforcement to managers and staff will add to perceptions of conflict. A leadership team that does not respect its members, deal with conflict constructively, or use effective communication is creating a dysfunctional organization.

Before resolution of conflict can begin, the cause of the conflict must be identified. There are different types of conflict—conflict within a person or a group, between groups, or between organizations. There are different causes of conflict at work, including organizational structure, goal incompatibility, competition for scarce resources, task interdependencies such as work shared between departments, and integration of roles. Group dynamics are a frequent source of conflict because people come with their own set of values, history, and expectations. Ethnic and cultural diversity of the nursing workforce can also lead to conflict, as well as to differing communication styles.

From my perspective as a consultant, conflict is overfeared and undervalued. Conflict happens every day to each of us. It is a part of life—from the moment we wake up in the morning to when we go to bed. We experience and handle many different types of conflict. When I had my carpet cleaned recently, the man from the cleaning company arrived late and was rude and unfriendly. When he entered my house, he asked me why I was wasting my money cleaning such an old and ugly carpet. This was not a great way to start off our business encounter!

Sometimes supervisors use work-scheduling tactics that cause conflict for employees. Scheduling you on days you attend school or when you don't have child care undoubtedly will cause friction. The source of the conflict can't always be removed, but how you handle it is crucial to resolution. Many nurses are ineffective at managing conflict.

For Your Toolkit

Conflict is overfeared and undervalued.

Why are nurses ineffective when confronted with conflict in the workplace? Most nurses would rather avoid conflict altogether than deal with whatever issue causes the tension. I'm not sure what makes conflict so difficult for nurses. It may be lack of training in managing conflict. For some, undoubtedly, fear of the conflict-resolution process is the hard part. For others, conflict may always be seen as a negative personal issue and therefore to be avoided at all costs. For the profession of nursing as a whole, conflict has been avoided or glossed over and not dealt with. This has caused many formidable and difficult issues to be endlessly debated but never resolved.

Consider the touchy and sensitive topic of appropriate educational preparations for nursing. Discussion has been going on for at least 40 years over whether entry into nursing practice should be at the associate degree or baccalaureate level, and there is still no education statement defining entry into practice for nursing. Various professional organizations and states have created their own statements, but no universal set of expectations yet exists.

According to Bernard and Walsh (1996), conflict is a normal, unavoidable part of human relationships and can be a growth process if people learn how to manage it effectively. From the perspective of Hitt et al. (1986), although each conflict situation has unique causes, most can be traced to four major sources: goal incompatibility, competition for scarce resources, task interdependencies, and organizational structure.

Consider this situation. You are working in an emergency department as a manager, and the hospital CEO tells you at a management meeting that he has invited all the physicians from a neighboring hospital to start using your department for their emergency patients. You are already short-staffed and do not have enough beds for emergency patients because patients waiting for admission are in at least half of your beds. How excited will you be to have more patients in your ER? This is a great example of goal incompatibility.

If you are short of nurses and count on the nurse staffing office to provide you with employees, what happens when six units each want a nurse, and there are only four nurses scheduled as floats? This becomes a conflict over scarce resources. If you work in the intensive care unit on the night shift, and the admitting department determines that they will no longer staff an admissions clerk on the night shift, you are affected by that decision. If the admissions manager makes that decision without talking to the ICU manager, and the nurses in ICU are expected to create admission documents on all new admits to ICU, you will have a conflict over task interdependencies. If you are a manager called to an emergency management meeting at 4:00 p.m. on a Friday afternoon and the CEO doesn't show up because he is leaving on a trip with his family, you will likely feel conflict over the organizational structure and lack of respect in your facility.

Conflict exists when two or more parties (individuals, groups, or organizations) differ with regard to facts, opinions, beliefs, feelings, drives, needs, goals, methods, values, or anything else (Bernard & Walsh, 1996). The conflict produced by the differences between these parties creates tension and discomfort. Because of the discomfort, most people view conflict as negative and something to be avoided if possible. There are managers and executives who perceive that shouting at a subordinate is the way to solve conflict. This is not the case, and besides that, is highly unprofessional. I have a colleague who recently told me that she cannot remember the last time she and her boss (a vice president) had a calm discussion about disagreements. Her boss yells at her whenever they disagree. Not only is that approach extremely unprofessional, it is a huge staff-retention issue!

Disagreement between groups about their goals can create conflict, especially if the accomplishment of one group's goals prevents the other group from achieving its goals. If a hospital wants to change how units are staffed and a nurse bargaining unit from a labor union files a grievance, the union group can inhibit the reconstructed staffing. This becomes incredibly frustrating for everyone involved, even when the objections to a new strategy are valid. Consider something like electronic medical records. If you see benefits for you in *not* implementing electronic medical-records technology, then you will feel conflict if your unit is to adopt an electronic record-charting system. Competition for scarce resources is an all-too-common theme for conflict in today's healthcare institutions. Dollars, people, space, and time are all in short supply.

If you depend on another unit or department to help you achieve your goals, conflict will occur if that department achieves a goal that negatively affects your department. As in the previous example, closing the admitting office after midnight may be seen as a great cost-saving measure by the admitting department, but as a major inconvenience for the ER or ICU night-shift staff.

Most organizational structures also cause conflict. Differing goals, roles, and viewpoints between managers and subordinates, or project managers and operations staff, are common and often difficult to resolve. In this era of constantly increasing healthcare costs and ever-decreasing healthcare dollars, there is more conflict than ever!

Some nurses may be unprepared to handle conflict. Many nurses are women, and in some cultures, women may not be brought up to deal with conflict. While this is not universally true, men tend to be socialized to see conflict as a usual occurrence in life, not as a personal attack or unusual situation. This may be partially due to men having more exposure to competitive sports, where conflict reigns on the field, but friendships endure once the game is over.

The other challenge for nurses in dealing with conflict is the issue of accountability. Sometimes staff nurses perceive that they do not have any decision-making power, or they expect someone else to handle a problem. But many patient-care improvements have been initiated by staff nurses who decided to change some aspect of care they felt strongly about. Family at the bedside during a code blue and creating blood sugar management protocols in a critical care unit are examples of nurses effectively managing conflict to create positive change.

Change almost always causes conflict. Conflict is part of the natural change process. Although individuals can resist the current changes we are seeing in health care, the impetus for change comes from both outside (e.g., the federal government) and inside the healthcare industry. Conflict results from implementing changes such as insurance-covered well-baby care or pain management documentation requirements. Conflict can resolve differences, clarify issues, and promote unity when managed effectively. To avoid conflict is to eliminate the possibility of defining goals, discussing issues, and designing a unifying philosophy about the issue.

For Your Toolkit

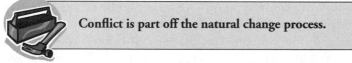

Conflict is part off the natural change process.

Conflict can also be about power. If you are a leader who implements change, conflict will inevitably be a by-product of that change. For a leader to use his/her power effectively, s/he must deal with the conflict in order for the change process to take place. To avoid conflict is to ignore the power of leadership. Surrendering power creates ineffective leaders and limits change potential when healthcare organizations need it.

Conflict in and of itself is not bad. It creates tension and makes people feel uncomfortable. Ignoring conflict and tension is what causes poor problem resolution, frustration, and defensiveness. Conflict is often seen as negative. The negativity is not inherent in conflict itself, but rather comes from tension caused by not handling the original issue or because of inappropriate methods of dealing with the issue (remember the screaming VP). Nurses often fear conflict because the tension it creates makes them less articulate, and the increased stress, workload, and time demands make conflict feel personal.

Conflict does enhance advocacy. Above all else, nurses continually strive to be advocates. Patients, families, and the underserved are the recipients of that advocacy. Handling conflict effectively allows patient advocacy to flourish. Not to deal with conflict limits patient advocacy and intervention effectiveness.

There are two ways to deal with conflict. One way is to use conflict resolution techniques. There are different types, including team-building, sharing perspectives nondefensively, attempting to focus on cooperative goals, transition management, education, and communication. Conflict resolution seeks a solution that satisfies all parties involved in the conflict. Rarely is it possible to satisfy all the needs of everyone involved. Some compromises are usually made to reach agreement. Legal arbitration is another type of conflict resolution.

The more common way to deal with conflict is through conflict management, which implies a conscious effort to deal with the conflict as well as the issue and control the problem. It does not guarantee to satisfy all involved, but attempts to meet as many needs as possible in determining a solution (Bernard & Walsh, 1996).

There are numerous issues that enter into a conflict situation. The values, goals, resources, and beliefs of the people involved will affect their willingness to compromise. Past relationships between conflicting parties are also important. If you have no respect for or do not trust your adversary, chances are you will not be committed to managing the conflict.

Nurses apply different strategies to conflict situations. The first choice is often to deny that the conflict exists. This causes no change in the conflict situation at all. If denial doesn't work, some nurses try to ignore conflict. This may relieve the tension initially, but the relief is usually short-lived. Ignoring conflict causes relationships to further deteriorate, and people will keep feeling bad. Suppressing conflict may be why people think of it as negative and destructive.

While difficult, it is much easier in the long run to deal with conflict head on. Confrontation means letting the other party know you disagree and being willing to discuss the issues, using collaboration, arbitration, problem-solving, or compromise. Many nurses who deal with conflict get stuck in the confrontation and never get to the discussion phase.

Not dealing with conflict is the single most limiting factor in resolving nursing issues at both the local and national levels. The nursing profession has yet to be comfortable with the idea that conflict is a valuable process, and that creative dissonance is beneficial to addressing changing issues. Instead of dealing with conflict up front, nursing groups tend to take sides according to their special interests. No formal confrontation takes place, and as a result, the profession is perceived as divisive and splintered in its beliefs and goals. Although there has been some unity on dealing with the nursing shortage, many other nursing issues are still unresolved.

Physicians are usually more comfortable dealing with conflict than nurses. They certainly have just as many issues on which to disagree, but physicians are able to duke it out behind closed doors and come out with a united stance for their profession. I remember being in an interdisciplinary hospital meeting with both physicians and nurses on the committee. Two physicians got into a yelling match over a specific patient protocol. They argued most of the meeting. When the meeting was over and they were walking out the door, they were discussing their next opportunity to meet for a golf game. Clearly, their conflict was not personal, and did not encroach on their personal relationship.

Nurses could learn from that approach. We could be so much more powerful in dealing with nursing and healthcare social-policy issues if the profession were willing to get down and dirty to resolve its differences, before airing its dirty laundry and splintered decisions in public. As a profession, we tend to look as though the right hand doesn't know what the left hand is doing when it comes to such important intraprofessional issues as educational entry into practice, instead of arbitrating our conflicts and developing a unified stance to share with patients and the public.

The formation of the Federal Nursing Commission for the Institute of Medicine Study on Nursing Staff in Hospitals and Nursing Homes is a classic example of not dealing with conflict and going public with the issues before discussion. Chances are no commission would have been needed and almost $1 million in federal funds could have been saved if nursing representatives had dealt beforehand with perceptions and conflicts over staffing, patient-care outcomes, and nursing injuries. I had the privilege of providing testimony at the hearings on this topic and heard the chairman share a similar perspective about the formation of the commission.

Conflict will always have to coexist with nursing. Nurses will continue to disagree on issues fundamental to the profession and critical to patient advocacy. Resolving conflict takes a strong stomach and the willingness to be uncomfortable. Nurses need to learn that differing opinions are not unusual or bad, and that dissonance fosters creativity, innovation, and collaborative outcomes. Nurses need to stop being afraid of conflict and start learning to use it.

Chapter 10
Professional Advocacy

Nurturing Our Young

There are important functions in being a nursing advocate. It is our professional responsibility and part of being of service to perform these functions throughout our career.

- **Nurture those who come after you**. Nurses are famous for "eating our young." That is such a disturbing phrase, but so true. Let's change it to "nurturing our young." It is our responsibility to coach and mentor nurses less experienced than we are. Be kind to nursing students and new grads. You never know when *they* might end up taking care of *you*!
- **Feed the machine.** Talk about your career as a nurse and encourage others to join the profession. Participate in the career days at your local schools and volunteer to talk about nursing in your community.
- **Be an RN 24/7.** Identify and introduce yourself as a nurse whenever you meet a new person. Role-model professional conduct, clothing, and behavior whenever you are in public. It is tough to be depicted as a bimbette if you never act like one.
- **Let go of old issues.** We don't have to agree on everything to work together as a profession. The proper credentials for entry into nursing practice are not a silver bullet issue. We need to advocate for the profession and for each other.

- **Cultivate your experiences and skills.** Seek out opportunities to learn and experience new things. Every skill you acquire gets added to the personal career toolkit that you take with you from job to job. It can never be too full!
- **Become a lifelong learner.** Continue to take classes and advance your nursing knowledge. Commit to expanding your learning and long-term career development.
- **Use staff to their maximum potential.** It doesn't matter whether you are a manager or not. Chances are you work with someone that you delegate tasks to. Encourage them to expand their knowledge. Ensure you expect the best they can be and give them tasks that allow that behavior to emerge.
- **Nurture yourself emotionally and spiritually.** Because nursing is about being of service, remember to take care of yourself. Balance your life; feed your soul and your heart so you can continue giving to others.

For Your Toolkit

Experienced nurses must nurture those who come after them!

Nurse Retention

Nursing retention is the responsibility of *every* nurse. There are plenty of innovative strategies suggested by nursing executives, school directors, and faculty. There are different answers for different regions of the country, but we all need to focus on the same goal. Start looking at ways to increase nursing faculty positions and hire qualified individuals in your local community. Joint appointments of nursing managers and clinical staff to faculty positions is one way for hospitals and schools of nursing to partner. Part-time and shared faculty positions will increase enrollment of students and eliminate waiting lists. Nursing faculty need assistance with creating clinical faculty opportunities with local hospital nursing staff. Local nurse administrators can be used as paid guest lecturers. Ask your local hospitals to sponsor skills labs through regional hospital organizations.

For Your Toolkit

Nursing retention is the responsibility of *every* nurse.

Nurse staffing ratios and a deepening nursing shortage require solutions and strategies different from those used in the past. Although there is no one magic recipe to increase the number of student slots in nursing programs, there is one simple answer for college administrators and chancellors. Get started. Step up to the plate and do something! Nurses in both service and academia stand ready to assist but cannot do it without college and university chancellor impetus and input to expand educational capacity.

Healthcare facilities need to commit to several strategies to assist with reversing the nursing shortage in their geographic regions. Effective strategies include the implementation of magnet characteristics as outlined in The Magnet Recognition Program®. This program was developed by the American Nurses Credentialing Center to recognize healthcare organizations that provide the very best in nursing care and uphold the tradition within nursing of professional nursing practice.

The program also provides a vehicle for disseminating successful practices and strategies among nursing systems. The Magnet Recognition Program® is based on quality indicators and standards of nursing practice as defined in the American Nurses Association's *Scope and Standards for Nurse Administrators* (2003). The Magnet designation process includes the appraisal of both qualitative and quantitative factors in nursing.

Additional retention strategies include using foreign-trained nurses in U.S. hospitals. There is a decreasing trend to recruit foreign nurses as replacement staff, as being too expensive. However, there are foreign-trained nurses currently residing in the United States. The Board of Registered Nursing (BRN) in most states usually approves foreign nurses to apply for national RN testing (NCLEX) if they have completed obstetrics and psychiatric course work and clinical practice in the United States. To accommodate foreign nurses who currently reside in the United States, local community colleges can put them on wait lists for obstetrics and psychiatric nursing. When there's an opening, a foreign-trained nurse can be allowed to fill it.

Offering RN residencies to new graduate nurses upon hiring has been demonstrated as the best retention strategy by far (Gates & Rubano, 2004). Other focuses include an expansion of compressed salary grids and offering retention bonuses instead of sign-on/recruitment bonuses. Hospitals can host job-shadowing and tour days at facilities for high school and college students considering a nursing career. It has been demonstrated by several research studies that facilities providing formal education and valuing and compensating nurse preceptors and mentors have more satisfied employees and higher retention rates.

Retention strategies must also be specifically cultivated for the Boomer nurses. As they enter their fifties, many Baby Boom–era nurses can no longer cope with clinical bedside care. Creating and offering other employment opportunities within hospitals for nurses no longer able to manage the physical demands of bedside clinical nursing would go a long way to keeping Boomer nurses working instead of retiring. Using Boomer nurses for coaches, mentors, preceptors, and educators would let them provide valuable experience to new nurses who need compassionate and kind oversight.

Facilities can implement shorter shift options, including 4- to 6-hr shifts, as many older nurses cannot handle 12-hr shifts physically. Job-sharing or flexible or self-scheduling options are also nurse-retaining options.

Hospitals can also provide preretirement information sessions to discuss reassignment options. These nonclinical options could include case management, patient advocacy, education, quality improvement, or mentoring. Keeping older nurses in patient-care settings as mentors is a valuable resource for less experienced nurses and increases retention of both older and newer nurses. Healthcare systems may want to evaluate the feasibility of using a deferred pension fund jointly with employment, as public-service agencies have done throughout the country. Police and fire services facing massive retirements from employees hired after the Vietnam War developed deferred retirement options and plans. These plans, called DROP programs, allowed police and firefighters to retire from their positions if they had 20 or more years of service. They could then reapply for the same job, earning both a salary and pension at the same time. This strategy encouraged many police and firefighters to remain in the workforce instead of retiring. Most plans have a maximum enrollment time of five years, but that still helps with retention of important public service staff.

Facilities could consider hiring older nurses as RN retention specialists. Their roles/responsibilities could include meeting with older nurses, facilitating problem-solving, and being empathetic listeners. They would serve as mediator and mentor resources. In addition, they could try to get nurses back who left because of personal concerns and by creating innovative solutions for older nurses. Nurses in this type of role can save registered nurses while limiting vacancies. It's win-win for the healthcare facilities that embrace these types of retention ideas. The older nurses remain employed and the hospital improves staffing with experienced nurses.

Healthcare facilities also need to remember how important for retention is having effective and competent nurse managers. Fifty percent of employee satisfaction comes from their relationship with their bosses (Kaye & Jordan-Evan, 2002). Research shows that the quality of the relationship between a boss and subordinate is a primary predictor of intention to remain in a job or facility (Thomas, 1994).

An investment in strengthening an organization's leaders—from senior executives to middle managers to team leaders—pays off in all sorts of ways, but particularly in attracting and retaining employees (Buckingham & Coffman, 2001). Those hospitals that have measures to hold managers accountable for retention tend to experience lower turnover rates. Accountability measures include incorporating retention efforts in managers' performance appraisals, bonuses for taking action related to achieving a qualitative or quantitative change in the turnover rate, and periodic review of employee satisfaction in the manager's specific service area (Abrams, 2002).

The bottom line is that retention must be the new emphasis in healthcare facilities. Recruitment strategies must continue, but not to the exclusion of retaining competent nurses who want to keep working. Nurses must be seen as what they truly are—a precious resource and mainstay of hospital care.

For Your Toolkit

Retention must be the new emphasis in healthcare facilities.

Public Perception of Nursing

I did a program for the American Association of Critical Care Nurses (AACN) National Training Institute a few years ago. My task was to talk about the public perception of nursing. I struggled to prepare for this one-hour talk. After much soul-searching, I realized my presentation came down to three questions:

- What is the public perception of nurses?
- What do we, as nurses, want it to be?
- How do we change the problematic perceptions?

Part of the role of a nurse is to be an advocate for the profession. Most nurses are terrific patient advocates but rarely consider expanding that advocacy to the public perception of nursing. When was the last time you saw a negative portrayal of nursing? What did you do about it? My guess is that we can all remember negative media portrayals of nurses—in television sitcoms and popular magazines. Nurses portrayed as sexy bimbettes in short, tight uniforms, deep cleavage, and garter belts are my personal pet peeve.

What are the positive and negative perceptions of nurses in your community? What images and behaviors contribute to those perceptions and why? Why do they exist? What do you want the public to see? How will you change those public perceptions to ones that would benefit the nursing profession? What can be done to adjust public perceptions when warranted?

I don't have a lot of answers to these questions. What I do know is that it is up to every nurse to combat negative media portrayals of nursing. One of the ways to do that is to realize that we are in the public eye 24/7. At the grocery store. At the bank. At a nightclub or PTA meeting. When you say you are a nurse, people have a higher level of expectation about your behavior. Whether that is fair is up for debate. However, I believe that the public expects us to meet certain standards of behavior, just as they do police and firefighters.

Numerous studies have shown that nursing is the most trusted profession. We have demonstrated behaviors in the past to warrant those perceptions. I'm not quite

For Your Toolkit

It is up to every nurse to combat negative media portrayals of nursing.

sure where the gap is between being the most trusted profession and looking like a bimbette in a weekly sitcom. I don't pretend to have the answer to that problem either. What I do believe is that it is our individual responsibility to highlight positive attributes of nursing whenever we can.

- Participate in a career fair at your child's school.
- Volunteer for a blood pressure screening or to give flu shots in your neighborhood.
- Write letters to your newspaper editor about relevant nursing topics.

There are many ways to respond and represent nursing as a profession in a positive light. How you do that depends on where you live and your personality. Highlighting the benefits and features of the nursing profession can be a great reminder to us of what is great about our profession. It also gives us a chance to educate people about the complex leadership role we play in the healthcare system. It doesn't matter what you do. Just do something positive for nursing.

Nursing Survival Strategies During Turbulent Times

Nurses need survival strategies during turbulent times (see Table 10-1). Every nurse deals with difficulties in a healthcare organization. With the evolving nursing shortage and other challenges to health care, there are more and more occasions when you feel that you are barely surviving. Here are some strategies for survival during those tough times:

- Understand right-sizing of management and workers.
- Eliminate duplication of tasks and people.
- Crosstrain whenever possible.
- Eliminate fragmentation and departmental barriers.
- Minimize nonproductive time.
- Determine ways to move services to customers and patients.
- Find ways to measure and reward customer satisfaction and quality.
- Streamline patient processes, systems, and documentation.
- Be seen as a leader/supporter of the organizational mission and values.
- Epitomize the characteristics of an indispensable nurse.

TABLE 10-1   Risks and Rewards of Using Survival Strategies

Risks	*Rewards*
Inability to be positive all the time	Employment
Increased stress	Empowerment seized
Lack of security	Increased self-confidence
Ambiguity	Increased value to your organization
May be seen as traitor by colleagues	Personal growth
Feel caught in the middle/isolated	Opportunities for innovation
Crisis-oriented mentality	Expanding horizons and job choices
Changing relationships	Pride
Failure	Professionalism

Traditional behaviors and socialization of nurses also exist. These perceptions are often reality. I list them here to identify that reality without judgment:

For females

- Be dependent.
- Take care of others.
- Be there 24/7.
- Be nice.
- Don't be selfish.
- Be collaborative, even at your expense.
- Be warm, loving, nurturing.
- Don't bother anyone.
- Don't say "no."
- Don't get angry.
- Be thin, gorgeous, and have great clothes.
- Keep family traditions.
- Learn to read others and anticipate their needs (codependence!).
- Always cooperate, no matter what.
- Don't act smarter than boys.
- It is okay to cry if you are upset.

For males

- Be independent.
- Be aggressive.

- Express anger, but no other emotions.
- Never cry.
- Keep your feelings to yourself.
- View power and control as career success.
- Know that the female role is to nurture males.
- Regard home as just a place to relax with no accountability.
- Be direct and straightforward.
- Be goal-oriented and future-oriented.
- Know you are smarter than women and let them know it.
- Give directions.
- Be well built, muscular, and not fat.

Nursing Means Being of Service to Others

The real essences of nursing, as of any fine art, lie not in the mechanical details of execution, nor yet in the dexterity of the performer, but in the creative imagination, the sensitive spirit, and the intelligent understanding lying back of these techniques and skills. Without these, nursing may become a highly skilled trade, but it cannot be a profession or a fine art. All the rituals and ceremonials which our modern worship of efficiency may devise, and all our elaborate scientific equipment will not save us if the intellectual and spiritual elements in our art are subordinated to the mechanical, and if the means come to be regarded as more important than ends. (Robbins, 1996)

Nursing is a service field. Whereas the care and tasks we perform for patients are highly technical and sophisticated, the nursing role is about being of service. Patients (as well as physicians) are the customers and there is a responsibility for serving the customers to the best of our ability. (Do not mistake this concept for taking verbal or physical abuse from physicians. That is not the same thing.)

Customer service is about persuasion, influence, being courteous, honoring patients' feelings/needs, being present for the patient both inside and out, listening, interpreting nonverbal cues, and using intuition.

Being of service also means dealing with angry patients, families, staff, and physicians. There are numerous changes that occur in a healthcare setting that affect front-line staff. Some staff members can roll with the changes and not take them personally. Others have more difficulty separating their personal feelings from changes in the organization. These folks tend to get angry and take it out on whoever they work with most closely.

For Your Toolkit

Nursing is about being of service.

Being of service is stress-producing and exhausting. Be sure you take care of yourself, as outlined in the Chapter 2 section on balancing your life. It is important to let go of work and patient-care issues after hours and find ways to take care of your body, mind, and soul. The alternative to not taking care of yourself is burnout. There has been much written about nursing burnout. It is preventable. Be caring and an advocate for yourself as you would for a patient. Don't deny the need you have to have a balanced life, emotional stability, and a centered, peaceful soul. Learn ways to monitor your own health. Honor your feelings and physical sensations. As my dear friend Katheryn Kray Ponce says, "When you have had enough, you'll know." That way you can do something to change things. Keep in mind that when you feel bad, it is bad, and you need to take care of yourself.

Graciousness Is Mandatory

We all know how it feels to be treated rudely at a meeting, have someone not follow up as expected or promised, or when someone takes advantage of us as a professional contact. No matter what happens to you—mergers, acquisitions, downsizing, or layoffs—graciousness is mandatory. Rude behavior and unprofessional etiquette have no place in the work setting.

For Your Toolkit

Graciousness is mandatory.

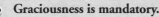

When you meet someone new, make eye contact and say hello. When you are in a room full of people, be sure your attitude is one of meeting everyone, as opposed to "What can you do for me?" Make sure you meet people because of inviting eye contact, not because you are shopping for important people. Make sure you have effective listening skills. Keep in mind that active listening is more than just not talking. There are lots of resources available you can use to enhance your listening skills if you frequently find yourself asking people to repeat themselves.

If you promise to assist or get back to someone, leave a voicemail or email with the information requested within a few days. To make someone wait longer is sloppy and unprofessional. Develop your own system to keep track of the business cards you get so they are not lost or forgotten. I usually write notes to myself on the back of business cards reminding me of how I met that person, what their children's names are, and the name of their secretary. The notes will help you remember important information as well as remember when to follow up.

Abuse in the Workplace

I am disappointed to report that as an employee, consultant, and Monster.com expert, I have heard about many incidents of on-the-job abuse by physicians, co-workers, supervisors, and patients. These incidents run the gamut from verbal abuse to throwing an operating room light fixture. Abuse of any sort is a very serious issue and should not be tolerated. Nurses sometimes become accustomed to abuse, and therefore it is ignored, avoided, or excused. Many nurses think they are powerless to combat abuse, or they perceive that no one in their organization really cares about it. You do have some options to take care of yourself and avoid abusive situations.

Almost all organizations have specific policies against harassment, abusive behavior, and hostile work environments. These policies are very strict, so familiarize yourself with the policy in your facility and the reporting process. You must also immediately report verbally any case of abuse to your supervisor. Depending on the circumstances, you may also need to submit a written report of the incident. If your supervisor does not respond or dismisses the incident, report it again through your human resources department.

Keep personal written records of the event and your reporting attempts. Keep an extra copy of that documentation at home, in what I like to call a hot file. That way, if anything happens to the work copies, there are others available. Use your hot file to document any potentially difficult or illegal incident that occurs in the workplace, including abusive behavior. Be sure to also follow your facility's required official documentation processes. Document whether the incident was isolated or ongoing, what occurred, the date, time, witnesses, who said what to whom, and what actions you took.

If the abuser is a manger who oversees others, that makes things a bit more complicated, but no more tolerable. When a manager is abusive, other supervisors and co-workers may choose to ignore or tolerate the situation. When bad behavior is overlooked, that behavior is supported and encouraged at some level—even if we don't mean to do so. In the event of an encounter with an abusive manager or supervisor, immediately call others to the scene to witness the behavior. There is strength in numbers, and you may be able to persuade your colleagues to join forces to stop the abuse.

It is all too common to hear of a physician screaming at a nurse about not being able to read illegible orders, not accepting a patient because the unit is full, or not being contacted when a patient is unstable. In my experience, abusive physicians are far more common than abusive nurses. My worst experience was having a physician scream at me about being incompetent as a director in front of the patient, the family, and several employees. Because he was so loud, every one on the unit heard his ranting. I decided that day that I would not let his behavior go unreported. I told the physician that it was clear to me he was very angry. I said I was unwilling to be spoken to like that, and when he calmed down I would be happy to meet with him about his concerns. Then I did the hardest thing of all—with my heart in my throat, I turned around and walked back to my office some distance away. Amazingly enough, he stopped yelling, finished up with the patient, and came to talk with me about 30 minutes later. His concerns were actually quite valid. It was his approach that was totally unacceptable. I did report his behavior through the medical staff reporting mechanisms, and he apologized to me and the staff. As far as I know, he never did it again to any other nurse in that facility.

The next time you are approached by a screaming physician, think about stopping the behavior for your sake, as well as for your co-workers'. You might attempt to confront the physician in private and inform him/her you do not wish to be spoken to in that manner, and advise him/her that you will be forced to report him/her to the medical director or department chair—whatever your policy dictates. You may also ask for an apology, although in my experience this tends to inflame these sorts of people even more.

You could also provide the offending physician, your supervisor, and the medical director or chair with a copy of at least one of the several articles written in the past several years about physicians' abusive behavior being a contributing factor to the nursing shortage. (See the sidebar "Articles on abuse.") I'm sorry to report there are a lot of them listed on the Internet.

Encourage your facility to adopt a physician code of conduct. When physicians understand that their behavior is contributing to the severe shortage of nurses in this country, most are happy to participate in the solution instead of being part of the problem. Create a committee composed of nurses, physicians, and administrators to develop a code of conduct, a physician abuse policy, and the mechanisms to curtail this type of behavior in your facility.

For Your Toolkit

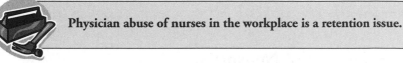

Physician abuse of nurses in the workplace is a retention issue.

The other group that tends to get abusive toward nurses is patients. I have had two experiences of this in my clinical career and both times were very scary. I had a patient in the ER break a glass IV bottle (yes, it was in those days) and threaten to kill

Articles on abuse

http://www.findarticles.com/p/articles/mi_m0FSL/is_3_74/ai_80159514
http://www.usnews.com/usnews/health/articles/020617/archive_021640.htm
http://xnet.kp.org/permanentejournal/winter04/pal.html
http://healthcare.monster.com/nursing/articles/verbalabuse/
http://www.nursingcenter.com/library/JournalArticle.asp?Article_ID=278949
http://www2.nurseweek.com/Articles/article.cfm?AID=14548

me with the jagged edge of the broken bottle. He was high on PCP, and the police were summoned. I ended up on the floor with him on top of me screaming. Fortunately, I wasn't hurt and the police responded quickly, but it was frightening. The other incident involved a father whose child died in ICU and could not contain his anger at the death of his only son. He threatened all the nurses who cared for his son with a gun. He calmed down quickly and never touched anyone, but the staff was really shook up.

Patients who attempt to assault nurses are dangerous and should be dealt with immediately. Employers are responsible and legally accountable to make responsible efforts to protect workers from workplace hostility. If you are assaulted by a patient, secure yourself and the other patients. Most facilities have a security code page for operators to use. Once the situation is controlled, report the event to your supervisor verbally and prepare a written report as well. Submit a report to the patient's physician. It may be that a patient who throws things or attempts to assault physically a nurse has a psychiatric disorder.

Most facilities have rules and policies about abusive behavior, but the reporting of these events is not common. Enforcing the rules usually only occurs when an incident comes up, so many nurses are not aware of the process before an event. Many nurses have learned to tolerate abuse, which only perpetuates the problem. Less tolerance of abusive behavior in the workplace will slowly force behavior to change. Protect yourself and your colleagues by taking appropriate action when these events occur. Taking care of yourself reflects your sense of your value as a human being and improves the workplace for everyone.

The Importance of Networking

Networking with other professionals is a process of creating links to obtain information, influence, and power. It is the process of exchanging information between strategically placed individuals who have access to ideas and other people (Turner, 1996). Networking is what makes people become connectors. Connectors are people that link ideas together between groups (Gladwell, 2004). Knowing connectors is valuable to your career, and using them well is priceless!

Nurses rarely recognize the value of using a professional network to enhance their careers. Some folks believe that asking for help means that they cannot do it on their own. There is nothing wrong with asking for help to achieve something. Folks who enjoy coaching and mentoring actually like being asked for help. If you have received value from being mentored, coached, or from using a network, be sure you offer it to others. It is up to those of us with experience to assist nurses coming along behind us so they too can be successful. It is not only a way to be of service, but part of our professional responsibility.

For Your Toolkit

> **Knowing connectors is valuable to your career, and using them well is priceless!**

The process of developing contacts and networking will assist you in accomplishing career goals, in problem-solving, and in advancing your career. It has often been said by management gurus that 75% of job offers come from networking (*not* from answering ads for interviews). This fact demonstrates that networking with other professionals is critical to your career success. Networking can be done in social situations, with family and friends, or at business meetings. It requires a conscious commitment of time, energy, and resources.

Networking is a long-term strategy for professional and career advancement. The rewards do not come quickly, and the benefits often take years to be realized. I once met a hospital administrator during an interview for a job I really didn't want, and spoke to her about my career goals. I shared what I wanted to do, and how I thought I could get there. She kept my business card and called me two years later when she had the kind of job I wanted. I worked with her for several years and still keep in contact.

Creating these linkages and networking with professionals is an active practice. It cannot be accomplished by default. You must dedicate energy and schedule time to do it. I find my most successful networking takes place over meals. It is relaxing to meet someone in a restaurant and talk with them about my goals. The value of the advice I get always outweighs what I paid for our meal. (If you invite someone to eat out with you for the purpose of networking, always pick up the tab.)

Networking can help you accomplish professional goals if you identify your own career goals and share them with mentors and coaches. You must create, initiate, and cultivate contacts. You must identify existing networks of colleagues and appropriate methods to achieve your goals and career advancement. Networking requires effort and thought on your part. If you do not put in the time and energy, you will not have a successful outcome.

Some folks are unclear on what constitutes networking. These activities are all part of active networking:

- Make phone calls just to chat—even when you don't need anything.
- Talk with colleagues about open positions you think they might be interested in or industry news (not gossip) that could be helpful to them.
- Promptly return phone calls from colleagues, especially if they request information from you.
- Write thank-you notes to colleagues for information or advice they have shared with you.
- Phone a colleague to ask for assistance in solving a problem.
- Invite colleagues or contacts out for lunch.

Strategies for successful networking include participation in a professional organization and subscribing to at least one professional journal/magazine. This kind of investment in your future will also assist you in deciding if you need further education, specialized training, or more subscriptions. It is important to keep up to date and informed in your specialty and about healthcare changes.

We have all been on the receiving end of a networking nightmare. Examine your own networking etiquette to see if you need to make some changes. It is inappropriate to network with the attitude "How can you help me?" You know the type. They scan name tags to see who will be useful to talk to and skip past those whose job titles seem uninteresting. Meet someone because of your inviting eye contact. It's tacky to shop only for important people.

When you first meet someone, don't blab on with self-importance. Practice a short introduction that states who you are and what you do. Try not to give just your job title, as if it explains everything. Job titles mean different things in different industries, so be specific.

Create a system for following up with people you meet. Design a filing system to keep track of the business cards you receive. Put notes on the back that will help you recall important information or remind you to follow up. Use voicemail, email, or a personal note to contact someone to whom you promised to respond. It's tacky to fail to contact someone, so always keep your promise.

Join at least one business organization, so you can begin building a reputation as a doer or a donor or both. You will be seen as someone who is serious about your career, your contacts, and your industry and not just a short timer. Be sure to send a thank-you note or make a thank-you call when someone has helped you. Doing so sends the message that you are gracious and not just a taker. Being gracious makes people want to help you again.

Don't wait until you have a crisis to start networking. Most folks wait for some drastic change in their professional life to make contact. A layoff or relocation can cause panic enough. Build a web of contacts *before* you need them, and when things are going well. Be sure to network with those people who are just starting out. It is tempting to network only upward, but you never know where they will be in a few years. That is especially true in health care.

Being available to network is crucial. If you are always too busy or never follow through, colleagues will stop making plans with you. To network successfully, you must be visible in the nursing community. To be visible takes time and energy. As you develop networks, mentors, and coaches, remember to say "thank you" for what you learn and for information that is shared—and never break a confidence or pass along private information.

Political Advocacy

Many healthcare issues that affect our communities are also social policy issues. Nurses are in a unique position to educate politicians about health issues. It is important for every nurse to become politically active.

> A healthy population is one of our nation's most important assets. To protect this asset, health care must be at the forefront of our society's consciousness. Without coherent state and national health care policies, the health of our communities and the existence of our hospitals are in jeopardy. (Association of California Nurse Leaders [ACNL], 1995)

Political influence is necessary to direct state and federal legislation that affects the operation of our healthcare delivery system. Providing knowledge about health and populations in the political process is an important role for caregivers. Because nurses have strong connections to their community and are employed in all parts of the healthcare continuum, they become crucial to influencing state and federal legislators as volunteer political advocates.

As a nurse, you have both the skills and expertise to educate legislators and citizens who are served and employed in your community. Politics and healthcare delivery systems get more interrelated as pressures for cost-effective, accessible, and quality

For Your Toolkit

Every nurse should be a political advocate for nursing.

healthcare services become part of the political agenda. Federal, state, and local fiscal management problems have necessitated greater government involvement in health care to control spending for public healthcare programs. The government must also assure that the fiscal limitations on healthcare providers do not deny access to care for people who need it.

Other factors are also changing the healthcare environment, in tandem with changes in public healthcare programs. The number of uninsured and underinsured persons has steadily climbed, adding more to already financially strained hospitals in the form of uncompensated care. An aging population, higher labor costs, new technologies, and labor shortages are additional factors aggravating the current healthcare situation.

Get informed about healthcare policy issues in your state and community. Learn about the legislative process. Reference materials specifically for nurses on healthcare policy advocacy are available from many professional nursing organizations, including the American Nurses Association, American Association of Critical Care Nurses, and the Association of California Nurse Leaders. Participate in public meetings and hearings on important issues. Write letters or make phone calls to your local legislators. Consider providing testimony at committee hearings on proposed bills. Who knows better than a nurse what patients' needs are?

As nurses you must become active participants in the legislative process. Influencing and changing the future of health care by educating lawmakers can make a difference. The need for grassroots support and advocacy has never been more important. You must contribute time and energy to the legislative process at a grassroots level in order to exert control over your destiny.

Chapter 11
Creating Your Nursing Future

"A 'turned-on person' has a vision of self and knows who they are,
has abundant energy and helps others discover their identity."

—AUTHOR UNKNOWN

Future Trends in Nursing

One of my favorite quotes is from the managed-care guru Paul Gann: "It is easy to come up with new ideas; the hard part is letting go of what worked for you two years ago, but will soon be out of date" (LaVally, 1999). It has never been truer for nursing practice than right now at the beginning of a new millennium.

In the past, the architecture of nursing has been based on a foundation of patient advocacy and achieving maximum beneficial outcomes for each patient. The framework of nursing care for patients included specialization of services, fragmented components of care, a narrow focus with minimum flexibility, and an us versus them mentality. Nursing has taken direction from other professions in terms of work tasks. Nurses have allowed other disciplines to dictate their scope of practice and role. We have designed our role around ancillary staff, such as clinical dieticians, respiratory therapists, physical therapists, and occupational therapists. This has caused us to give away pieces of the nursing process because of the constant

195

need to bend to the expectations of other disciplines. This framework is no longer compatible with the direction of the healthcare industry.

Several environmental factors are affecting the future of nursing practice:

1. Diversity—changing demographics in states' populations, the diversity of the nursing workforce, and public views of health care and healthcare policy issues.
2. Age—the impact of an aging population on healthcare systems, financing of health care, demand for nurses, an aging nursing workforce, and the development of new healthcare services.
3. Technology—the impact of global technology on roles and practice of nursing.
4. Workforce—challenges in healthcare workforce supply, demand, education, and role definition.
5. Healthcare financing—the impact of increasing costs and financing on delivery systems, community-based healthcare programs, and practice roles for nurses.

To meet the needs of our nation for the future, the nursing profession must change the framework in which care is provided. The architectural foundation remains the same. Patient advocacy and maximum beneficial care outcomes will continue to drive the way we provide care. However, we must eliminate much of the intraprofessional infighting that has kept us from achieving our goals and finding ways to affect fundamentally the health of our nation.

For Your Toolkit

The nursing profession must change the framework in which care is provided.

The framework we build for our future practice must be based on specific nursing roles as well as on integration of services, have a community-wide focus, include flexibility and cross-training of nursing staff, be committed to lifelong learning and professional development, have the mindset of us helping them, and have one focused, professional voice with which we change care practices to meet the needs of all our patients.

To achieve this new architecture and framework for nursing practice, additional changes must be made across the profession in the next 20 years. We need to expect an exponential and accelerated rate of change compared to past decades. Nursing education will be vastly different. Students will take prenursing courses online. Nursing programs will use multimedia and onsite clinical experiences like human simulation labs. An internship at the end of school and a residency at the beginning of new graduates' first year will be required.

Nurses will be everywhere, affecting healthcare in every feasible location—churches, schools, homeowners' associations, shopping malls. They will be seen as chronic-care coaches and managers. Patients will see physicians only when their conditions change. Nurses will be perceived as highly skilled, caring, and well-educated professionals. Replaced by the roles of clinician, coach, educator, and entrepreneur, the handmaiden image of the traditional nurse will finally pass away.

Nurses will be culturally competent with additional advanced practice skills in leadership, education, and supervision. They will be information gurus and spend much of their time absorbing and explaining information to others. Because of this enhanced nursing role, and the continued nursing shortage, the demand for licensed vocational/practical nurses and unlicensed assistive personnel will continue to rise.

The nursing workplace will be transformed. Staggered and part-time shifts will be the norm. Roles like retention coordinator and master preceptor will be created for older, experienced nurses. Clinical staff nurses will also be faculty in local nursing schools. Patient care will be monitored from nurses' homes. There will be no paper and no needles, and searchable electronic medical records and patient histories will be available throughout the United States.

Retention instead of recruitment will be the healthcare focus. The priority will shift to keeping nurses in the workforce, especially Boomer nurses. New retention strategies will be identified and implemented, using out-of-the-box thinking. Significant pension plans, paid education sabbaticals, and extended vacation time will be the norm.

Scheduling will be cafeteria style by which staff RNs will pick what works best for them. Positions will be thought of in terms of worked hours per pay period or month, and staff will pick a plan that works for them. Self-scheduling will be the norm, and salaries will reflect bonuses for weekend and holiday commitments.

There are some challenges to this kind of optimal professionalization and self-determination of nursing practice. These challenges include regulation of nursing practice by nursing organizations juxtaposed with the self-directed autonomy of nurses. Unionization of professional nurses versus self-governance of nurses will become a hot debate by the end of this current decade. There will be a wide diversity of nursing values that may overshadow shared beliefs and collaborative strategies for the profession. There will continue to be intraprofessional conflicts related to boundary management of what belongs in nursing practice and what is and what is not the realm of other practitioners. There will be more focused dialogue on nursing education differentiation (ADN, BSN, and MSN) and agreement on what the minimum educational foundation for professional practice should be. This will likely be an ongoing dialogue, with changes over many years.

The preferred future for nursing will require specific leadership strategies. These strategies will include autonomy for professional practice and career development and a knowledge-based foundation for practice. Nurses will develop leadership skills and competencies, and work intensively to improve the public perception of nursing. The use of evidence-based practice, driven by nursing research and outcomes-focused measurements for nursing and patients, will be commonplace.

Nurses will work in a self-governed workforce in a shared-governance model. Labor unions will have less impact on staffing ratios and use because this will be determined by the nurses themselves. This will require both professional and workplace influence on nursing practice. There will be social and community activism on health-policy-related issues. All of these strategies will mandate a lifelong learning environment for practicing nurses.

The role of the registered nurse in the future will be as a director and coordinator of care, not just a task performer. Nurses will become the choreographer of care for patients. Nurses will have an expanded practice with a redirected focus toward wellness. They will function in a community-based model using a case-management approach to provide care along the health–illness continuum. Nurses will continue to be routinely recognized as the work-task redesign experts. They will maintain basic skills and core competencies.

All these changes will require great transition-management skills. Nurses will need to create strategies for "making the incredible credible and the impossible possible," according to Richard Brock, RN, MN, Director of Medical Surgical Nursing at Good Samaritan Hospital, Los Angeles. Acknowledge your uniqueness and revel in keeping that intact. Don't try to cope alone; use your circle of support—friends, spouse, significant others, colleagues. This will help you manage your stress. Remember what your mother told you, but thrive on how things are changing so you can survive!

Creating Your Personal Nursing Future

Only you can determine the kind of professional nurse you want to be. It is easy to be passionate about a profession that gives you so many job and career choices. Nursing forces you to be the best you can be, no matter what your role. As Ruth Ann Terry, RN, MPH, executive officer of the California Board of Registered Nursing, says, "Nursing is a fabulous exciting career without boundaries" (Hugg, 2005). It is difficult for the general public to grasp that nurses—not physicians—are the fulcrum of health care. The nursing shortage has escalated the problems of a broken healthcare system. If nurses weren't crucial to the system, things wouldn't have become worse during the nursing shortage.

Lifelong learning throughout your nursing career will put you on the path to excellence. Life is about learning, and learning is about change. You must do both to carve out your personal future in nursing. If you lack awareness of changing circumstances or do not have an attitude that embraces change, your professional growth will be stunted. Lifelong learning complements the professional growth that comes with self-conscious experience (Deleonardi, 2005). Nurses committed to lifelong learning for their own professional development will have an exciting future in nursing.

For Your Toolkit

Life is about learning, and learning is about change.

Suzanne Gordon (2005) talks about the state of nursing in this country. Ms. Gordon is not a nurse but has observed and assessed our profession in great depth. She believes we are a profession on the brink. She believes it is up to the 2.7 million of us whether we create nursing's finest hour or worst hour in the next few years. We have the power to make or break health care right now—and for years to come. Each one of us has a responsibility as a professional nurse to secure care for our nation's population as well our profession's future. We hold the keys to changing systems and processes. Be sure you use your influence to enhance care and the profession in a positive way.

Using your nursing influence to enhance care is really about being a leader in society and using leadership skills. Dr. Warren Bennis is an internationally recognized management and leadership guru. As the chairman of the Leadership Institute at the University of Southern California, he defined leadership in one sentence: "A leader is one who manifests direction integrity, hardiness and courage in a consistent pattern of behavior that inspires trust, motivation and responsibility on the part of the followers who in turn become leaders themselves"(Johnson, 1998).

Bennis believes that people want four things from their leaders. I believe nurses have all of them. "First, direction and meaning; second, trust; third, a sense of hope and optimism—some way of investing in the future; and finally, they want results. These are the four things that all people want." Leaders have to provide a sense of purpose to give direction and meaning. They have to be authentic to provide trust. They have to enable and develop authentic relationships, and they have to have a sense of hardiness in order to provide a sense of optimism and hope.

Leaders are people who generally believe things will work out well and that one can influence the circumstances of one's life—an expectation for success. Leaders also have a bias toward action, as well as courage and the ability to act. Most nurses I have known have these characteristics inside their nursing souls.

Use your own nursing soul every day, whatever role you are in. Generate a sense of purpose in your organization that honors nursing and the patients you care for.

Spread your vision and purpose throughout the institution and give fellow nursing colleagues a sense of meaning. Keep reminding people what is important. Encourage people to be straightforward and honest. Leadership is really about being empathetic and caring about people. Leadership is being candid all the time. Given the complexity of life and health care, nurse leaders must take decisive action and some risks.

Nurses are leaders. Nurses are also winners at what they set out to accomplish. Start leading and exhibiting behaviors of a winner as soon as you finish this book. Nursing is a career for life and a way of life. Support the renaissance of our profession by mentoring kindly those who come after you and showing them the ways of the future. Demonstrate the qualities of a winner as you plan your career goals and your future. Good luck!

The Winner

The Winner is always a part of the answer.
The Loser is always a part of the problem.
The Winner always has a program.
The Loser always has an excuse.
The Winner says, "Let me do it for you."
The Loser says, "That's not my job."
The Winner sees an answer for every problem.
The Loser sees a problem for every answer.
The Winner says it may be difficult, but it's possible.
The loser says it may be possible, but it's too difficult.
A Winner listens.
A Loser waits until it's his turn to talk.
When a Winner makes a mistake, he says, "I was wrong."
When a Loser makes a mistake, he says, "It wasn't my fault."
A Winner says, "I'm good, but not as good as I could be."
A Loser says, "I'm not as good as lots of other people."
A Winner feels responsible for more than his job.
A Loser says, "I only work here."

—Author unknown

References

Abrams, M. (2002, March). "Employee Retention and Turnover: Holding Managers Accountable." *Trustee.* 55 (3), T1.

Advance News magazine. (2005). "Advancing Your Career." Retrieved 7/12/05 from www.advanceweb.com.

Advisory Board Daily Briefing. (2001, April 9). "Severe Nursing Shortage Is Threat to Patient Care." Retrieved April 2001 from www.advisory.com.

Allen, Jane E. (2001, May 7). "U.S. Nurses Not Alone in Their Frustration." *Los Angeles Times.* p. B10.

American Nurses Association. (1993). *Nursing's Agenda for Health Care Reform.* Washington, D.C.: ANA Publishing.

———. (2002). *Call to Action.* Washington, D.C.: ANA Publishing.

———. (2003). *Scope and Standards for Nurse Administrators.* Washington, D.C.: ANA Publishing.

AONE. (2002, September). "Say What? What California Nurses Say About Working." *Nurseweek/AONE Study.* Retrieved 8/16/05 from www.aone.org.

Association of California Nurse Leaders. (1995). *ACNL Resource Guide for Political Action.* Aliso Viejo, CA: American Association of Critical Care Nurses.

Bach, David. (2005, September). "Get That Raise." *Working Mother.* p. 52.

Barada, Paul W. (2005). "How Do You Sell Yourself When You Don't Have Much to Sell?" Retrieved 7/13/05 from http://content.monstertrak.monster.com/resources/archive/jobhunt/toughsell/.

Barnes, C., and Sutherland, S. (1999). *Survey of Registered Nurses in California, 1997.* Sacramento, CA: Board of Registered Nursing.

Benefits of Becoming a Magnet-Designated Facility. Retrieved 8/16/05 from www.nursingworld.org/ancc/magnet/benes.html.

Benner, P., Tanner, C.A., & Chesla, C.A. (1996). *Expertise in Nursing Practice: Caring, Cinical Judgment and Ethics.* New York: Springer.

Bensing, K. (2005, August 8). "No Stone Unturned." *Advance for Nurses.* Southern California edition. p. 11.

Bernard, L., and Walsh, M. (1996). *Leadership: The Key to Professionalization of Nursing.* New York: Mosby.

Bernstein, A., and Craft-Rozen, S. (1995, March/April). "Why Don't They Just Get It?" *Executive Female.* pp. 33–37.

Beverly Health and Rehabilitation Services. (1990). *Supervisory Training Modules.* Rancho Cordova, CA: Author.

Beyers, Marjorie. (1996, February 5). "The Value of Nursing." *Hospitals and Health Networks.* p. 52.

Borg L. (2000, May 10). "We Have Been Giving Until It Hurts—Nursing Losing Patience with Overtime." *Providence (R.I.) Journal-Bulletin.* p. 1B.

Bradley, Carol. (2002, March). "The Nursing Shortage: Facilitating Partnerships Between Service and Education." Garden Grove, CA: CACN Fall Conference. Data from Deans and Directors Survey.

Brown, Steve. (2001, May 21). "Congress Spotlights Nursing Shortage, Rural Wage Index Workforce Issues." *AHA News.* 37 (20).

Brownstein, M. (2000). *Coaching and Mentoring for Dummies.* Foster City, CA: IDE Books Worldwide.

Brzezicki, Lisa. (2005, Aug. 22). "Caring for the Caregiver." *Advance for Nurses,* Southern California edition. p. 9.

Buckingham, M., & Coffman, C. (2001). *First, Break All the Rules: What the World's Greatest Managers Do Differently.* New York: Simon & Schuster.

Buerhaus, P. (1998). "Is Another RN Shortage Looming?" *Nursing Outlook.* 46 (3), 103–108.

———. (1999). "Is a Nursing Shortage on the Way?" *Nursing Management.* 30 (2), 54–55.

———. (2000, June 14). "Implications of an Aging Registered Nurse Workforce." *JAMA.* 83 (22).

Buerhaus, P.I., & Staiger, D.O. (1997). "Future of the Nurse Labor Market According to Health Executives in High Managed Care Areas of the United States." *Image—The Journal of Nursing Scholarship.* 29 (4), 313–318.

Buerhaus, P., Staiger, D.O., and Auerbach, D.I. (2000). "Implications of an Aging Registered Nurse Workforce." *Journal of the American Medical Association.* 283 (22), 2948–2987.

California Board of Registered Nursing. (2000). *Annual School Report,* 1998–99.

California Strategic Planning Committee for Nursing/Colleagues in Caring. (1999, January). "Competency Based Differentiated Roles Nursing Practice Model." University California, Irvine.

ChooseNursing.com. (2004). *Paying for Nursing School.* Retrieved February 2006 from http://www.choosenursing.com/paying/financialaid.html.

Coffman, J., Spetz, J., Seago, J.A., Rosenhoff, E., & O'Neil, E. (2001, January). *Nursing in California: A Workforce Crisis.* San Francisco, CA: Workforce Initiative and the UCSF Center for the Health Professions. Retrieved 2/2001 from http://futurehealth.ucsf.edu/CWI/nursingneeds2.html.

Cowles, Luke. (2005, March 7). "First Impressions." *Advance for Nurses.* p. 23

Davis, Carolyn, Ed. (1996, August). *Nursing Staff in Hospitals and Nursing Homes: Is It Adequate?* Washington, D.C.: National Academy Press, National Institute of Medicine.

Deleonardi, Bette. (2005, September 5). "Lifelong Learning." *Advance for Nurses.* pp. 17–22.

Denning, E. (2000). *Out of the Crisis.* Cambridge, MA: MIT Press.

DeRitis, S. (2004, April 26). "New Opportunities within Healthcare Informatics." *Advance,* p. 31.

Dick, Thom. (2005, June). "Listening: Defusing the Angry Employee." *Emergency Medical Services.* p. 28.

Donaho, Barbara, Ed. (1996, August). *Celebrating the Journey: A Final Report on Strengthening Hospital Nursing.* Washington, D.C.: National Academy Press.

Drucker, P. (2001). *The Essential Drucker.* New York: Harper Collins.

Erwin J. (1999, March 29). "Aging Out? Will the Rising Age of O.R. Nurses Lead to a Shortage?" *Nurseweek.*

Fackelmann, K. (2000, June 15). "Study Predicts Nursing Shortage." *USA Today.*

Fischman, Josh. "Nursing Wounds." *U.S. News & World Report.* Retrieved 8/02 from www.usnews.com/usnews/health/articles/020617/archive_021640.htm.

Gaffin, Norma Mushkat. (2004). "Recruiters' Top 10 Resume Pet Peeves." Retrieved 7/13/05 from http://resume.monster.com/articles/petpeeves/.

Gates, Polly, & Rubano, Joan. (2004, Fall). *Executive Coaching or Mentoring: Which Way Should You Go? DirectLink Newsletter.* Sacramento, CA: Association of California Nurse Leaders. p.1.

Gladwell, Malcolm. (2004). *Tipping Point.* New York: Little, Brown.

Gordon, S. (2005). *Nursing Against the Odds.* Ithaca, NY: Cornell University Press.

Goulette, Candy. (2005, June 13). "Under Their Wings." *Advance for Nurses.* Southern California edition. pp. 38–39.

Health Resources and Services Administration. "National Sample Survey of Registered Nurses." Retrieved 2/2001 from www.nurseweek.com/nursingshortage.

Hill, Linda. (1998). "Maximizing Your Influence." *Working Woman.* pp. 21–24.

History of Men in Nursing. Retrieved 8/16/05 from www.geocities/Athens/forum/6011/sld006.html.

Hitt, M., Middlemist, R., & Mathis, R. (1986). *Management Concepts and Effective Practice,* 2nd ed. Houston, TX: West Publishing.

Hollander, Jim. (2005, June 26). "Onboard Medical Facilities Have Cruise Passengers Covered." *Los Angeles Times.* p. L3.

Hugg, Alicia. (2005, July 4). "Forging Ahead." *Nurseweek.* pp. 8–10.

Hunsacker, P.L., and Allesandria, A.L. (1980). *The Art of Managing People.* New York: Simon & Schuster.

Johnson, James. (1998). "Warren Bennis, Chairman, The Leadership Institute." *Healthcare Executive.* Retrieved 7/15/05 from www.ache.org/pubs/hcexecsub.cfm.

Kaye, B.L., & Jordan-Evan, S. (2002). *Love 'Em or Lose 'Em: Getting Good People to Stay.* San Francisco, CA: Benett-Koehler Publishers.

Kennedy, M.M. (1996, September/October). "When Your Career Is Sidelined." *Executive Female.* pp. 33–35.

Komisarjevsky, C., and Komisarjevsky, R. (2004). *Peanut Butter and Jelly Management: Tales from Parenthood Lessons for Managers.* New York: Amacom.

Krueger, Richard. (1994). *Focus Groups: A Practical Guide for Applied Research.* Thousand Oaks, CA: Sage Publications.

LaVally, R. (1999). "Laws of the Century: 200 Significant Statutes and Constitutional Amendments of the 20th Century." California Senate Office of Research. Retrieved July 2005 from http://www.sen.ca.gov/sor/reports/REPORTS_BY_SUBJ/LAWS_OF_CENTURY.HTP.

Lewin, K. (1947). "Group Decision and Social Change." In Newcomb, T., Hartely, E., eds., *Readings in Social Psychology.* New York: Holt, Rinehart and Winston.

Lichtenberg, Ronna. (2005, July/August). "Designing a Future That Fits." *More.* pp. 60–64.

Lipow, Valerie. (2005). "Interviewing 101." Retrieved 7/13/05 from http://hourlyandskilled.monster.com/retail/articles/retailinterviewing/.

Lumsdon, Kevin. (1995, December 5). "Faded Glory." *Hospitals and Health Networks.* pp. 31–36.

Lyon, Mary. (1998). "The ABCs of Pursuing Higher Education in Nursing." *Nurseweek Career Fair.*

Malugani, Megan. (2005). "Legal Nurse Consulting." Retrieved 7/12/05 from http://featuredreports.monster.com/nursing05/legal/.

———. (2005). "Up-and-Coming Nurse Niches." Retrieved 7/11/05 from http://featuredreports.monster.com/nursing05/niches/.

Marks, Mitchell. (1994). *From Turmoil to Triumph.* Boston: Lexington Press.

Mayer, G. (1997, July/August). "The Impact of Managed Care on Hospital Nursing." *Best Practices and Benchmarking in Healthcare.* pp. 162–167.

McGraw, Phil. (2005, June). Column. *Oprah.* Chicago: Harpo Productions. p. 31.

McGregor, D. (1960). *The Human Side of Enterprise.* New York: McGraw-Hill.

McLinden, Steve (2005). "Navigating Organizational Culture." *Nurseweek Pathways to Success.* pp. 102–105.

Mehallow, Cindy. (2005). "Nursing Careers Beyond the Bedside." Retrieved 7/10/05 from http://featuredreports.monster.com/nursing05/nonclinical/.

———. (2005). "Nursing Careers Beyond the Hospital." Retrieved 7/10/05 from http://featuredreports.monster.com/nursing05/nonhospital/.

Merritt, Jennifer. (2005). "Get-Ahead Strategies You've Never Heard Before." Retrieved 7/14/05 from http://reference.aol.com/onlinecampus/campusarticle?id=20050712200509990001.

Meyeroff, Wendy J. (2005). "Advance Your Nursing Career." Retrieved 7/12/05 from http://featuredreports.monster.com/nursing05/advancedspecialties/.

Miller, Judith. (1995, Summer). "Leading Nursing into the Future." *Harvard Nursing Research Institute Newsletter.* 4 (3), 5–7.

Mooney, Bette. (2005, July 11). "Resolving Conflicts." *Advance for Nurses.* Southern California edition. p.15.

Myss, Caroline. (2003). *Sacred Contracts.* New York: Three Rivers Press.

National Council of Nursing State Boards. (1997). "NCN Identifies Functional Abilities Essential for Nursing Practice." *Issues 97.* 18 (1), 8–9.

Noer, David. (1995, July/August). "After the Pink Slips." *Executive Female.* pp. 43–45.

Pew Health Professions Commission. (1995, Summer). "Healthy America: Practitioners for 2005." *Pew Health Professions Report.*

Porter, P. (2000, May 10). "Nomadic Nurses Fill Staffing Gaps." *The Columbus* (OH) *Dispatch.*

RN Scope of Practice. (2001). *California Business and Professional Code, Section 2725.*

RN Special Advisory Committee, State of California. (1990). "Meeting the Immediate and Future Needs for Nursing in California."

Robbins, Stephen. (1996). *Organizational Behavior,* 7th ed. Upper Saddle River, NJ: Prentice Hall.

———. (2002). *Organizational Behavior,* 10th ed. Hoboken, NJ: Prentice Hall.

Rossheim, John. (2005). "Nurses Who Teach." Retrieved 7/10/05 from http://featuredreports. monster.com/nursing05/professorship/.

Ruiz, M. (2000, Third Quarter). "Nursing Shortage." *Sigma Theta Tau International Honor Society of Nursing in Clinical Practice.* pp. 2948–2954.

Rundio, Al. (2005). "Ten Management Pearls for Success." *Nurseweek Pathways to Success.* pp. 24–25.

Russell, G. (2000, April 21). "Nursing Schools See Enrollment Steadily Shrink." Worcester, MA: *Telegram Gazette.*

Sechrist, K. et al. (1999, August). *Final Report.* California Strategic Planning Commission for Nursing.

Selis, S. (2000, June) "Where Have All the Nurses Gone?" *Healthcare Business.* 3 (4), 65–70.

Smith, Mike. (2005, June). "Beyond Competent." *Emergency Medical Services.* p. 42.

Spetz, J. (1996, October). "Nursing Staff Trends in California Hospitals: 1977–1995." Sacramento, CA.: Public Policy Institute of California.

Steefel, L. (2005, July 4). "Survey Shows First Real Positive Workforce Change." *Nurseweek,* p.15.

Stern, C. (1990). *Kaiser Foundation Hospital Graduate Nurse Handbook of Job Searching Techniques,* 4th ed. Oakland, CA: Kaiser Permanente Hospitals.

Stewart, M. (1998, March/April). "New Nursing Shortage Hits; Causes Complex." *American Nurse.* 30 (2), 14–18.

Stringer, Heather. (2005, August 29). "Turning Point." *Nurseweek,* p. 12.

Thomas, D. (1994, November/December). "Five Ways to Run Your Career Like a Business." *Executive Female.* pp. 37–40.

Turner, Susan Odegaard. (1995a, May). "Laid Off: Now What?" *Nursing.* pp. 94–95.

———. (1995b, January). "Stand Out or Lose Out!" *Nursing.* pp. 13–18.

———. (1996). *Transitions in Healthcare Series.* Aliso Viejo, CA: American Association of Critical Care Nurses.

———. (1998). *Transitions in Health Care Series,* 2nd ed. Aliso Viejo, CA: American Association of Critical Care Nurses.

———. (1998). *Has the Restructuring of Registered Nursing Roles in Hospitals Been Successful?* Doctoral dissertation. College of Business, University of Southern California.

———. (1999). *Nurse's Guide to Managed Care.* Gaithersberg, MD: Aspen Publishers.

———. (2000, April). "Regional Nursing Shortage Report." *RHORC.* p. 1.

Versant RN Residency. (2005). Retrieved 7/14/05 from www.versant.org.

Vogt, Peter. (2005). "Measure Your Soft Skills Smarts." Retrieved 7/13/05 from http://content.monstertrak.monster.com/resources/archive/jobhunt/softskills.

Warren, Rick. (2002). *The Purpose Driven Life.* Grand Rapids, MI: Zondervan.

Wilson, B. (1997). *Men in American Nursing History.* Retrieved February 2006 from http://www.geocities.com/Athens/Forum/6011/.

Woodward, Harry. (1994). *Navigating Through Change.* New York: Richard D. Irwin, Inc.

Worthington, Michael. (2004). "Top 20 Recruiter Pet Peeves About Resumes." Retrieved 7/12/05 from http://resumedoctor.com/.

Organizations and Web Sites*

Organizations

American Nurses Association
   http://nursingworld.org
Nurses for a Healthier Tomorrow
   http://www.nursesource.org
Nursing Economics
   http://www.ajj.com
National League of Nursing
   http://www.nln.org
The Forum on Health Care Leadership
   http://www.healthcareforum.org
Bureau of Labor Statistics
   http://www.bls.gov
American Hospital Association
   http ://www.aha.org
American Organization of Nurse Executives
   http://www.aone.org
American Association of Colleges of Nursing
   http://aacn.nche.edu

National State Boards of Nursing
   http://www.ncsbn.org
Allnurses.com
   http://allnurses.com
Choose Nursing!
   http://www.choosenursing.com
Johnson/Johnson site
   http://www.discovernursing.com
Monster.com
   http://www.monster.com
Health Career information
   http://www.healthprofessions.com
Health Career information
   http://www.healthcareers.com
Visa Information
   http://www.visalaw.com
Nursing Spectrum
   http://www.nursingspectrum.com

*Listing is not an endorsement, and URLs change from time to time.

209

National Student Nurses Association
  http://www.nsna.org
Links to nursing Web sites
  http://www.nursezone.com
Johnson and Johnson Nursing site
  http://www.choosennursing.com
Nurses for a Healthier Tomorrow
  http://www.nursesource.org/
Nursing Economics
  http://www.ajj.com
The Forum on Health Care Leadership
  http://www.healthcareforum.org
Bureau of Labor Statistics
  http://www.bls.gov
Nursing 2000
  http://www.nursing2000inc.org
Exceptional Nurse.com
  http://www.exceptionalnurse.com
Minority Nurses
  http://www.minoritynurse.com
Legal nurse consultants
  http://www.aalnc.org
Managed care nurses
  http://www.aamcn.org
Neuroscience nurses
  http://www.aann.org
Nurse anesthetists
  http://www.aana.com
Occupational health nurses
  http://www.aaohn.org
Office nurses
  http://www.aaon.org
Spinal cord injury nurses
  http://www.aascin.org
Specialties certifications
  http://www.nursingcertification.org
Political info on health care
  http://www.healthvote.org
Medical-surgical nurses
  http://medsurgnurse.org
Nurse practitioners
  http://www.aanp.org
Men in nursing
  http://www.aamn.org

Critical care
  http://www.aacn.org
Diabetic nurse educators
  http://www.aadenet.org
Association of California Nurse Leaders
  http://www.acnl.org
U.S. Senate
  http://www.senate.gov
U.S. House of Representatives
  http://www.houseofrepresentatives.gov
U.S. legislature
  http://www.legislature.gov

Career Transition

The Transition Network
  http://www.thetransitionnetwork.org
Ruby Slippers
  http://www.yourownrubyslippers.com
International Coach Federation
  http://www.coachfederation.com

Nursing Blogs

www.codeblog.com
http://mediblogpathy.blogspot.com
http://head-nurse.blogspot.com
http://deathmaiden.blogspot.com

Organizations

Accreditation Assn. for Ambulatory Health Care
9933 Lawler Ave.
Skokie, IL 60077-3708
Phone: (847) 676-9610
Fax: (847) 676-9628
E-mail: aaahc@mcs.com

AIDS Healthcare Foundation
1300 N. Vermont Ave., Suite 407
Los Angeles, CA 90027
Phone: (213) 662-0492
Fax: (213) 662-0196

AIDS Project Los Angeles
1313 N. Vine St.
Los Angeles, CA 90028
Phone: (213) 993-1600
Fax: (213) 993-1598

Alpha Tau Delta Natl. Fraternity for Professional Nurses
150 Cruickshank Drive
Folsom, CA 95630
Phone: (916) 984-9150

Am. Academy of Ambulatory Care Nursing
E. Holly Avenue, Box 56
Pitman, NJ 08071
Phone: (609) 256-2350
Fax: (609) 589-7463
E-mail: aaacn@mail.ajj.com
Web: http://www.inurse.com/~aaach

Am. Academy of Nurse Practitioners
Capitol Station/LBJ Building
P.O. Box 12846
Austin, TX 78711
Phone: (512) 442-4262
Fax: (512) 442-6469
E-mail: admin@aanp.org

Am. Academy of Pain Management
13947 Mono Way, Suite A
Sonora, CA 95370
Phone: (209) 533-9744
Fax: (209) 533-9750
E-mail: aapm@aapainmanage.org
Web: http://www.aapainmanage.org

Am. Academy of Pediatrics
141 Northwest Point Blvd., P.O. Box 927
Elk Grove Village, IL 60009-0927
Phone: (847) 981-7872
Fax: (847) 228-5097
E-mail: kidsdocs@aap.org

Am. Academy of Physical Medicine and Rehabilitation
1 IBM Plaza, Suite 2500
Chicago, IL 60611-3604
Phone: (312) 464-9700
Fax: (312) 464-0227
Web: http://www.aapmr.org

Am. Assn. for Health Education
1900 Association Drive
Reston, VA 20191
Phone: (703) 476-3437
Fax: (703) 476-6638
E-mail: aahe@aahperd.org
Web: http://www.aahperd.org/aahe.html

Am. Assn. for the History of Nursing
P.O. Box 90803
Washington, DC 20090-0803
Phone: (202) 543-2127
Fax: (202) 543-0724
Web: http://users.aol.com/nsghistory.aahn.html

Am. Assn. for Respiratory Care
11030 Ables Lane
Dallas, TX 75229-4593
Phone: (972) 243-2272
Fax: (972) 484-2720
Web: http://www.aavc.org

Am. Assn. for World Health
1825 K St. N.W., Suite 1208
Washington, DC 20006
Phone: (202) 466-5883
Fax: (202) 466-5896
E-mail: aawhstaff@aol.com
Web: http://www.aawhworldhealth.org

Am Assn. of Colleges of Nursing
1 DuPont Circle N.W., Suite 530
Washington, DC 20036
Phone: (202) 463-6930
Fax: (202) 785-8320
Web: http://www.aacn.nche.edu

Am. Assn. of Critical-Care Nurses
101 Columbia
Aliso Viejo, CA 92656
Phone: (800) 899-2226
Fax: (714) 362-2020
Web: http://www.aacn.org

Am. Assn. of Diabetes Educators
100 W. Monrow, 4th floor
Chicago, IL 60603
Phone: (800) 338-3633
Fax: (312) 424-2427
Web: http://www.aadenet.org

Am. Assn. of Health Plans
1129 20th St. N.W., Suite 600
Washington, DC 20036
Phone: (202) 778-3200
Fax: (202) 331-7487
Web: http://www.aahp.org

Am. Assn. of Healthcare Consultants
11208 Waples Mill Road, Suite 109
Fairfax, VA 22030
Phone: (703) 691-2242
Fax: (703) 691-2247
E-mail: consultahc@aol.com
Web: http://www.aahc.net

Am. Assn. of Homes and Services for the Aging
901 E St. N.W., Suite 500
Washington, DC 20004-2037
Phone: (202) 783-2242
Fax: (202) 783-2255
Web: http://www.aahsa.org

Am. Assn. of Legal Nurse Consultants
4700 W. Lake Ave.
Glenview, IL 60025
Phone: (847) 375-4713
Fax: (847) 375-4777
E-mail: info@aalnc.org

Am. Assn. of Neuroscience Nurses
224 N. Des Plaines, Suite 601
Chicago, IL 60661
Phone: (312) 993-0043
Fax: (312) 993-0362
E-mail: assnneuro@aol.com
Web: http://www.aann.org

Am. Assn. of Nurse Anesthetists
222 S. Prospect Ave.
Park Ridge, IL 60068-4001
Phone: (847) 692-7050
Fax: (847) 692-6968
Web: http://www.aana.com

Am. Assn. of Nurse Attorneys
3525 Ellicott Mills Drive, Suite N
Ellicott, ND 21043
Phone: (410) 418-4800
Fax: (410) 418-4805
E-mail: taana@assochq.com

Am. Assn. of Office Nurses
109 Kinderkamack Road
Montvale, NJ 07645
Phone: (201) 391-2600
Fax: (201) 573-8543
E-mail: aaofnurse@cyber.net

Am. Assn. of Poison Control Centers
3201 New Mexico Ave. N.W., Suite 310
Washington, DC 20016
Phone: (202) 362-7217
Fax: (202) 362-8377
Web: http://www.aapcc.poison.org

Am. Assn. of Retired Persons
601 E St. N.W.
Washington, DC 20049
Phone: (202) 434-3470
Fax: (202) 434-6483
E-mail: member@aarp.org
Web: http://www.aarp.org

Am. Assn. of Spinal Cord Injury Nurses
75-20 Astoria Blvd.
Jackson Heights, NY 11370-1170
Phone: (718) 803-3782
Fax: (718) 803-0414
E-mail: info@epva.org
Web: http://www.epva.org

Am. Assn. on Mental Retardation
444 N. Capitol St. N.W., Suite 846
Washington, DC 20001-1512
Phone: (202) 387-1968
Fax: (202) 387-2193
E-mail: aamr@access.digex.net
Web: http://www.aamr.org

Am. Cancer Society
1599 Clifton Road
Atlanta, GA 30329
Phone: (800) ACS-2345
Fax: (404) 329-5787
Web: http://www.cancer.org

Am. Chronic Pain Assn.
P.O. Box 850
Rocklin, CA 95677
Phone: (916) 632-0922
Fax: (916) 632-3208
E-mail: acpa@pacbell.net

Am. College of Allergy, Asthma, and Immunology
85 W. Algonquin Road, Suite 550
Arlington Heights, IL 60005
Phone: (847) 427-1200
Web: http://allergy.mcg.edu

Am. College of Health Care Administrators
325 S. Patrick St.
Alexandria, VA 22314
Phone: (703) 549-5822
Fax: (703) 739-7901
Web: http://www.acaca.org

Am. College of Nurse Practitioners
1090 Vermont Ave. N.W., Suite 800
Washington, DC 20005
Phone: (202) 408-7050
Fax: (202) 408-0902

Am. College of Nurse-Midwives
818 Connecticut N.W., Suite 900
Washington, DC 20006
Phone: (202) 728-9860
Fax: (202) 728-9897
E-mail: info@acnm.org
Web: http://www.acnm.org

Am. College of Preventive Medicine
1660 L St. N.W., Suite 206
Washington, DC 20036
Phone: (202) 466-2044
Fax: (202) 466-2662
Web: http://www.acpm.org

Am. Congress of Rehabilitation Medicine
4700 W. Lake Ave.
Glenview, IL 60025
Phone: (847) 375-4725
Fax: (847) 375-4777
Web: http://www.acrm.org

Am. Diabetes Assn.
1660 Duke St.
Alexandria, VA 22314
Phone: (703) 549-1500
Fax: (703) 549-6995
Web: http://www.diabetes.org

Am. Health Information Management Assn.
919 N. Michigan Ave., Suite 1400
Chicago, IL 60611
Phone: (312) 787-2672
Fax: (312) 787-9793
Web: http://www.ahima.org

Am. Heart Assn.
7272 Greenville Ave.
Dallas, TX 75231
Phone: (214) 373-6300
Web: http://www.amhrt.org

Am. Holistic Nurses Assn.
4101 Lake Boon Trail, Suite 201
Raleigh, NC 27607
Phone: (800) 278-2466
Fax: (919) 787-4916

Am. Lung Assn.
1740 Broadway
New York, NY 10019
Phone: (212) 315-8700
Fax: (212) 265-5642
E-mail: info@lungusa.org
Web: http://www.lungusa.org

Am. Nurses Assn.
600 Maryland Ave. S.W., Suite 100 W.
Washington, DC 20024-2571
Phone: (800) 274-4262
Fax: (202) 651-7001
Web: http://www.nursingworld.org

Am. Nurses in Business
P.O. Box 741384
Houston, TX 77274-1384
Phone: (713) 771-5016

Am. Occupational Therapy Assn.
4720 Montgomery Lane
P.O. Box 31220
Bethesda, MD 20824-1220
Phone: (301) 652-2682

Am. Pain Society
4700 W. Lake Ave.
Glenview, IL 60025
Phone: (847) 375-4715
Fax: (847) 375-4777
E-mail: info@painsoc.org

Am. Physical Therapy Assn.
1111 N. Fairfax St.
Alexandria, VA 22314
Phone: (703) 684-2782
Fax: (703) 706-8575
Web: http://www.apta.org

Am. Radiological Nurses Assn.
2021 Spring Road, Suite 600
Oak Brook, IL 60521
Phone: (630) 571-9072
Fax: (630) 571-7837
E-mail: arna@rsna.org

Am. Society for Parenteral and Enteral Nutrition
8630 Fenton St., Suite 412
Silver Spring, MD 20910-3805
Phone: (301) 587-6315
Fax: (301) 587-2365
E-mail: aspen@nutr.org
Web: http://www.clinnutr.org

Am. Speech-Language-Hearing Assn.
10801 Rockville Pike
Rockville, MD 20852
Phone: (301) 897-5700
Fax: (301) 571-0457
Web: http://www.asha.org

Asian and Pacific Islanders Am. Health Forum
942 Market St., 2nd Floor
San Francisco, CA 94102
Phone: (415) 954-9988
Fax: (415) 954-9999
E-mail: hforum@apiahf.org
Web: http://www.apiahf.org/apiahf

Assn. for the Education and Rehabilitation of the Blind and Visually Impaired
4600 Duke St., Suite 430
Alexandria, VA 22304
Phone: (703) 823-9690
Fax: (703) 823-9695
E-mail: aernet@laser.net

Assn. for Professionals in Infection Control, Epidemiology
1016 16th St. N.W., Sixth Floor
Washington, DC 20036
Phone: (202) 296-2742
Fax: (202) 296-5645
Web: http://www.apic.org

Assn. of Asian Pacific Community Health Organizations
1440 Broadway, Suite 510
Oakland, CA 94612
Phone: (510) 272-9536
Fax: (510) 272-0817
E-mail: info@aapcho.org
Web: http://www.aapcho.org

Assn. of Nurses in AIDS Care
1555 Connecticut Ave. N.W., Suite 200
Washington, DC 20036
Phone: (215) 321-2371

Assn. of Operating Room Nurses
2170 S. Parker Road, Suite 300
Denver, CO 80231
Phone: (303) 755-6300
Fax: (303) 750-3213
Web: http://www.aorn.org

Assn. of Pediatric Oncology Nurses
4700 West Lake Ave.
Glenview, IL 60025-1485
Phone: (847) 375-4724
E-mail: apon@amtec.com

Assn. of Rehabilitation Nurses
4700 W. Lake Ave.
Glenview, IL 60025-1485
Phone: (800) 229-7530
Fax: (847) 375-4777
E-mail: info@rehabnurse.org

Case Management Society of America
8201 Cantrell Road, Suite 230
Little Rock, AR 72227
Phone: (501) 225-2229
Fax: (501) 221-9068
Web: http://www.cmsa.org

Center for Science in the Public Interest
1875 Connecticut Ave. N.W., Suite 300
Washington, DC 20009-5728
Phone: (202) 332-9110
Fax: (202) 265-4954
E-mail: cspi@cspinet.org

Child Welfare League of America
440 First St. N.W., 3rd Floor
Washington, DC 20001-2085
Phone: (202) 638-2952
Fax: (202) 638-4004
Web: http://www.cwla.org

Children's Defense Fund
25 E St. N.W.
Washington, DC 20001
Phone: (202) 628-8787
Fax: (202) 662-3510
Web: http://www.childrensdefense.org

**Commission on Graduates of
Foreign Nursing Schools**
3600 Market St., Suite 400
Philadelphia, PA 19104
Phone: (215) 222-8454
Fax: (215) 662-0425

Family Violence Prevention Fund
383 Rhode Island St., Suite 304
San Francisco, CA 94103-5133
Phone: (415) 252-8900
Fax: (415) 252-8991
E-mail: fund@fvpf.org
Web: http://www.fvpf.org/fund

Hispanic Health Council
175 Main St.
Hartford, CT 06106
Phone: (860) 527-0856
Fax: (860) 724-0437
Web: http://www.hispanichealth.com

Hospice Assn. of America
228 7th St. S.E.
Washington, DC 20003
Phone: (202) 547-7424
Fax: (202) 547-3540
Web: http://www.nahc.org

Hospital Nurses Assn.
Medical Center E, Suite 375
211 N. Whitfield
Pittsburgh, PA 15206
Phone: (412) 687-3231
Fax: (412) 361-2425
E-mail: hnsfan@usa.pipeline

International Assn. for the Study of Pain
909 N.E. 43rd St., Suite 306
Seattle, WA 98105
Phone: (206) 547-6409
Fax: (206) 547-1703
E-mail: iasp@lock.hs.washington.edu

**Joint Commission on Accreditation of
Healthcare Organizations**
1 Renaissance Blvd.
Oakbrook Terrace, IL 60181
Phone: (630) 792-5000
Fax: (630) 792-5005
Web: http://www/jcaho.org

Natl. Alliance for the Mentally Ill
200 N. Glebe Road, Suite 1015
Arlington, VA 22203-3754
Phone: (703) 524-7600
Fax: (703) 524-9094
E-mail: namioffic@aol.com
Web: http://www.nami.org

Natl. Asian Pacific Center on Aging
1511 Third Ave., Suite 914
Seattle, WA 98101-1626
Phone: (206) 624-1221
Fax: (206) 624-1023

Natl. Assn. of Neonatal Nurses
1304 Southpoint Blvd., Suite 280
Petaluma, CA 94954
Phone: (707) 762-5588
Fax: (707) 762-0401
E-mail: nannmbrs@aol.com
Web: http://www.ajn.org/ajnnet/hrsorgs/nann

**Natl. Assn. of Nurse Practitioners in
Reproductive Health**
1090 Vermont Ave. N.W., Suite 800
Washington, DC 20005
Phone: (202) 408-7025
Fax: (202) 408-0902
E-mail: nanprh@aol.com

Natl. Assn. of Orthopaedic Nurses
401 N. Michigan Ave., Suite 2200
Chicago, IL 60611
Phone: (800) 289-6266
Fax: (312) 527-6658
E-mail: naon@smithbucklin.com

Natl. Assn. of School Nurses
P.O. Box 1300
Scarborough, ME 04070-1300
Phone: (207) 883-2117
Fax: (207) 883-2683
E-mail: nasn@aol.com

Natl. Assn. of Social Workers
250 First St. N.E., Suite 700
Washington, DC 20002-4241
Phone: (800) 638-8799
Web: http://www.naswdc.org

Natl. Black Child Development Institute
1023 15th St. N.W., Suite 600
Washington, DC 20005
Phone: (202) 387-1281
Fax: (202) 234-1738
E-mail: moreinfo@nbcdi.com
Web: http://www.nbcdi.org

Natl. Black Nurses Assn.
1511 K St. N.W., Suite 415
Washington, DC 20001
Phone: (202) 393-6870
Fax: (202) 347-3808
E-mail: nbna@erols.com

**Natl. Center for the Advancement of Blacks in
the Health Professions**
P.O. Box 21121
Detroit, MI 48221
Phone: (313) 345-4480

Natl. Council of State Boards of Nursing
676 N. St. Clair, Suite 550
Chicago, IL 60611-2921
Phone: (312) 787-6555
Fax: (312) 787-6898
Web: http://www.ncsbn.org

Natl. Council on Aging
409 Third St. S.W., Suite 200
Washington, DC 20024
Phone: (202) 479-1200
Fax: (202) 479-0735
E-mail: info@ncoa.org
Web: http://www.ncoa.org

**Natl. Council on Alcoholism and Drug
Dependence**
12 W. 21st St.
New York, NY 10010
Phone: (212) 206-6770, ext. 220
Fax: (212) 645-1690
E-mail: national@ncadd.org
Web: http://www.ncadd.org

Natl. Flight Nurses Assn.
216 Higgins
Park Ridge, IL 60068
Phone: (847) 698-1733
Fax: (847) 698-9407
E-mail: enainfo@ena.org
Web: http://www.ena.org

Natl. League for Nursing
350 Hudson St.
New York, NY 10014
Phone: (212) 989-9393
Fax: (212) 989-3710
Web: http://www.nln.org

Natl. Organization for Associate Degree Nursing
11250 Roger Bacon Drive, Suite 8
Reston, VA 20190
Phone: (703) 437-4377
Fax: (703) 435-4390
Web: http://www.noadn.org

Natl. Student Nurses Assn.
555 W. 57th St., Suite 1327
New York, NY 10019
Phone: (212) 581-2211
Fax: (212) 581-2368
E-mail: nsna@nsna.org
Web: http://www.nsna.org

Oncology Nursing Society
501 Holiday Drive
Pittsburgh, PA 15220
Phone: (412) 921-7373
Fax: (412) 921-6565
E-mail: members@ons.org
Web: http://www.ons.org

Respiratory Nursing Society
7794 Grow Drive
Pensacola, FL 32514
Phone: (904) 474-8869
Fax: (850) 484-8762
E-mail: rns@aol.com

Sickle Cell Disease Assn. of Am.
200 Corporate Point, Suite 495
Culver City, CA 90230-7633
Phone: (310) 216-6363
Fax: (310) 215-3722

Sigma Theta Tau International Honor Society of Nursing
550 W. North St.
Indianapolis, IN 46202
Phone: (317) 634-8171
Fax: (317) 634-8188
E-mail: stti@stti.iupui.edu
Web: http://www.nursingsociety.org

Society of Gastroenterology Nurses and Associates
401 N. Michigan Ave.
Chicago, IL 60611
Phone: (800) 245-7462
Fax: (312) 321-5194
E-mail: sgna@sba.com
Web: http://www.sgna.org

Society of Urologic Nurses and Associates
E. Holly Avenue, Box 56
Pitman, NJ 08071-0056
Phone: (609) 256-2335
Fax: (609) 589-7463
E-mail: suna@mail.ajj.com

United Ostomy Assn.
19772 McArthur Blvd.
Irvine, CA 92612-2405
Phone: (800) 826-0826
Fax: (714) 660-9262
E-mail: uoa@deltnet.com
Web: http://www.uoa.org

Visiting Nurse Assn. of America
11 Beacon St., Suite 90010
Boston, MA 02108
Phone: (617) 523-4042
Fax: (617) 227-4843

Wound, Ostomy, and Continence Nurses Society
1550 S. Coast Highway, Suite 20
Laguna Beach, CA 92651
Phone: (888) 224-9626
E-mail: membership@wocn.org
Web: http://www.wocn.org

Nursing

Nursing . . . a career not measured in years, but in moments. . . . A Victorian crazy quilt. A nursing career. What do they have in common? Rich fabric. Fragmented. Held together by heart and hand. Elaborately embellished with unforgettable moments. Fine art. Painstakingly expected. A work in progress, often unfinished. Chaotic yet controlled. And synergy . . . the whole is greater than the sum of its parts. In the end, we will not remember the years we spent in nursing. We will remember only the moments.

—Melodie Chenevert, RN

Index